Medicare and Medicaid

Recent Titles in the
CONTEMPORARY WORLD ISSUES
Series

Books in the **Contemporary World Issues** series address vital issues in today's society such as genetic engineering, pollution, and biodiversity. Written by professional writers, scholars, and nonacademic experts, these books are authoritative, clearly written, up-to-date, and objective. They provide a good starting point for research by high school and college students, scholars, and general readers as well as by legislators, businesspeople, activists, and others.

Each book, carefully organized and easy to use, contains an overview of the subject, a detailed chronology, biographical sketches, facts and data and/or documents and other primary source material, a forum of authoritative perspective essays, annotated lists of print and nonprint resources, and an index.

Readers of books in the Contemporary World Issues series will find the information they need in order to have a better understanding of the social, political, environmental, and economic issues facing the world today.

Medicare and Medicaid

A REFERENCE HANDBOOK

Greg M. Shaw

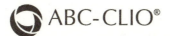

ABC-CLIO®

An Imprint of ABC-CLIO, LLC

Santa Barbara, California • Denver, Colorado

Library of Congress Cataloging-in-Publication Data

Names: Shaw, Greg M., author.

Title: Medicare and medicaid : a reference handbook / Greg M. Shaw.

Description: Santa Barbara : ABC-CLIO, 2021. | Series: Contemporary world issues | Includes bibliographical references and index.

Identifiers: LCCN 2020024080 (print) | LCCN 2020024081 (ebook) | ISBN 9781440873348 (hardcover) | ISBN 9781440873355 (ebook)

Subjects: LCSH: Medicare. | Medicaid. | Social medicine—United States.

Classification: LCC RA412.3 .S534 2021 (print) | LCC RA412.3 (ebook) | DDC 368.4/2600973—dc23

LC record available at https://lccn.loc.gov/2020024080

LC ebook record available at https://lccn.loc.gov/2020024081

ISBN: 978-1-4408-7334-8 (print)
      978-1-4408-7335-5 (ebook)

25 24 23 22 21   1 2 3 4 5

This book is also available as an eBook.

ABC-CLIO
An Imprint of ABC-CLIO, LLC

ABC-CLIO, LLC
147 Castilian Drive
Santa Barbara, California 93117
www.abc-clio.com

This book is printed on acid-free paper ∞

Manufactured in the United States of America

Preface

To the great extent Americans are ambivalent about government involvement in health care, a balanced account of health policy in the United States might begin like Charles Dickens' 1859 novel *A Tale of Two Cities*. "It was the best of times, it was the worst of times, it was the age of wisdom, it was the age of foolishness." Americans currently live during a time of remarkable technological advances in medicine that have rendered many debilitating or fatal conditions as relics of the past. Joint replacements and organ transplants have become essentially routine. American babies born as much as 10 weeks prematurely usually survive. The last wild case of polio was seen in the United States in 1979, before most Americans alive today were born. The survival rates for most types of cancer are higher than they have ever been.

However, Americans also spend far more on health care than people in any other country, and the United Sates spends a larger share of its overall wealth on these services than does any other nation. Despite this, the United States has only mediocre public health statistics to show for it. The American infant mortality rate places the United States behind most industrialized democracies. The same can be said about the rate of mortality amenable to health care, that is, the number of deaths that could be avoided with proper health care services. The politics surrounding health care is so conflicted that majorities of Americans not only support increased government spending on health but also disapprove of many of the recent proposals to extend insurance to more of the population. Medicaid has become the nation's primary way of paying for nursing home care, yet about one-quarter of the states have declined (as of 2020), on a partisan basis, to expand that program to cover more near-poor residents despite Congress's offer to pay 90 percent of the additional costs. Barely one-half of American adults hold a favorable view of the Affordable Care Act, yet neither political party has been able to muster the votes in Congress to significantly adapt the law to an ever-evolving health insurance landscape, other than to eliminate the controversial requirement that virtually all Americans should obtain health insurance and to delay the implementation of the tax on high-cost private insurance plans. Public opinion polls routinely show that most Americans believe government should do more to expand health insurance, but calls for Medicare for All receive distinctly mixed responses. Observers might be forgiven for concluding that Americans really don't know what they want in the way of health care policy.

That this book went to press during the worst pandemic in a century tragically added several other layers of importance to this conversation. In the view of many public health professionals, the U.S. health care system, as piecemeal as it is, was not particularly prepared for the onslaught of patients the COVID-19 virus has created. Not only should clinic and hospital staff not have to worry about shortages of things as basic as personal protective equipment, the insufficiency of intensive care beds and ventilators further highlighted the work to be done in order to create a world-class health care system. Beyond the equipment shortages, three other elements have stood out. First, the 9.1 percent of Americans who lack health insurance (as of early 2019) poses significant challenges not only for these nearly 30 million people who don't know how they would pay for services if the virus befell them but also for their medical providers. While the vast majority of providers want to be able to service all comers, the costs that will be passed on to those who are insured will be tremendous.

Second, COVID-19's disproportionate impact on less healthy persons has revealed how some of these co-morbidities, especially respiratory problems, are structured by race and class. To date, African Americans have suffered illness and death from the virus at a significantly higher rate than other groups. That they also account for more than their share of the uninsured population creates a recipe for outsized impacts. Finally, the dysfunction of many parts of Americans' health care discourse showed itself again during the spring of 2020 when a strong partisan divide emerged on questions of the severity of the pandemic and whether or not people should take it seriously, adjusting their lives accordingly. That Democrats and Republicans would resort to their party identification—displaying 30- to 40-percentage point spreads—to interpret a pandemic that, since spring 2020, has killed tens of thousands of Americans each month and has, as of this writing, cut short over 200,000 lives is nothing short of appalling (see the NPR/PBS/Marist poll of March 13–14, 2020). While it shouldn't be necessary to have to say it, protecting public health should not be a partisan matter. But the evidence says it is.

Medicare and Medicaid are thoroughly bound up in these debates. Together, these two massive federally sponsored programs account for approximately one-half of all health care spending in the United States. In 2018, Medicare supported 60 million Americans at a cost of $750 billion. That same year, Medicaid supported 75 million Americans at a cost of $597 billion. Of course, at its genesis neither program was envisioned to be so far-reaching. The expansion of Medicare, and to an even greater extent Medicaid, has involved a series of steps to help specific groups at particular moments in time—dialysis patients, individuals living with HIV/AIDS, pregnant women, young children, the working poor—instead of pursuing any sort of overarching, coherent strategy to get to universal coverage. As the saying goes, politics is the art of the possible, as opposed to the ideal, and the histories of Medicare and Medicaid certainly show this to be true.

The relationship between Americans, their health insurance, and their government is a tortured one. Over the past few decades, solid majorities of Americans have come to support Medicaid coverage for low-income and even middle-income people, support that has facilitated gradual expansions that have converted Medicaid into considerably more than the welfare medicine program it was originally designed to be. It is now the nation's third-largest payer for health care, behind private insurance and Medicare. At the same time, many Americans remain skeptical, even resentful, toward government involvement in health care. Opponents often invoke the specter of incompetent bureaucrats poised to interfere in the doctor-patient relationship, or a fear of "socialized medicine," or a "Washington takeover" of this sector. As the trope goes, if you like visits to the DMV, you'll love government health care. Prominent also is the complaint that Medicare and Medicaid are fundamentally broken entitlement programs, a critique that highlights the difficult-to-control costs for both federal and state governments. These deep conflicts over the public's perspectives of government involvement in health care have hobbled what could otherwise be constructive conversations about how to engineer a smarter set of financing and delivery systems. Instead, a rather unhealthy public discourse generally prevails.

This reference handbook offers an in-depth discussion of the two main government health care programs that together cover more than 135 million Americans, or nearly 40 percent of the population. Medicare, which covers persons who are either over age 65 or disabled, and Medicaid, which is limited to lower-income individuals and families, act as insurance that reimburses providers for medical goods and services. Because these programs cost tax payers hundreds of billions of dollars annually, and because of the life-line they provide to such a large portion of the population, the politics surrounding Medicare and Medicare are often highly contentious. Naturally, the persons enrolled and their families strongly want to preserve these means of health insurance and generally see them as an earned right. Medical providers often resent the low reimbursement levels paid by these programs, but they also recognize these payments as better than simply performing charity care. Policy makers struggle to find ways to pay for these very expensive programs. Taxpayers hold a mix of views, ranging from puzzlement about how these programs work to strong support, to concern about how federal and state budgets will cover the huge expenses of health care for an aging population.

Despite the frequent criticism of Medicare and Medicaid by politicians and others, these two programs, over the course of the past half century, have done tremendous good for many millions of people, young and old, poor and not, in-patient and out-patient. The peace of mind for the elderly envisioned by Medicare's architects in the 1960s has allowed generations of senior citizens to retire without undue worry about how they will meet their medical needs. This has gone a long way toward lifting the elderly out of financial distress and stands as one of the key achievements of the War on Poverty (Bailey and Danzinger 2013). For their part, many Democratic politicians and their followers have called for an expansion of Medicare to cover all Americans. As is often the case, exactly how such a proposal might work has not yet been fleshed out.

The lack of political agreement about the ideal scope of Medicare and Medicaid eligibility and service coverage has led each generation of policymakers to make what have been mostly minor adjustments—within the bounds of what is politically possible at the time—to these programs. For Medicare, the net effect has been to broaden the scope of services covered but not the types of persons eligible. It remains available only to those who are at least 65 years of age and to the long-term disabled. In contrast, the changes to Medicaid have broadened both the range of services covered and the eligible population, which now includes working-age persons of modest income who are not necessarily poor. One might think of these many changes across time as a very large and elaborate building that generations of architects have worked on. Each generation has its own idea of how the edifice should look, and each generation leaves its own imprint on the design, even if those ideas don't closely match what the original builders had in mind in 1965. Throughout the 1990s into the 2000s, various changes broke the bond that Medicaid traditionally had with welfare, expanding coverage for millions of modest-income children and adults. Without these changes, tens of millions of Americans would not have their present health insurance, and many thousands would die prematurely for lack of adequate care (more than already do). Most nursing homes would have to fundamentally curtail who they accept as patients. Hospitals and smaller clinics would have to dramatically alter their business models and alter their missions regarding how they try to care for all comers. Despite all their faults, Medicare and Medicaid are integral parts of the fabric of American health care.

Plan of the Book

Chapter 1 discusses the mid-20th century history of how Medicare and Medicaid came to be and the evolution of these programs up to the present. Emphasis is given to historical developments that have had the most powerful impacts on current Medicare and Medicaid policies and problems. Readers interested in exploring the policy history more deeply than space allows here will find suggested readings in chapter 6. Chapter 2 builds on this history by examining several of the current and near-term challenges to Medicare and Medicaid, ranging from high costs, under-performing ways to control those to long-term skilled nursing services, to prescription drug prices. Chapter 2 also considers a range of possible solutions, including many of those discussed in the run-up to the 2020 elections and those that are likely to persist as prominent issues for years to come. To help readers consider some of the implications of the policy challenges and possible solutions, chapter 3 consists of a series of essays from informed observers and participants who offer perspectives from interest groups, health policy scholars, medical providers, and beneficiaries. These observers offer diverse views that will challenge many readers to see government health insurance in a more complex way. Chapter 4 complements these contributed essays by surveying a range of important organized stakeholders, describing the work they have done recently to advocate for their positions. This will help readers to better understand current health politics. Chapter 5 presents a wide variety of facts and figures on the current programs for those interested in quantifying the demographic and financial impact that Medicare and Medicaid have on our country's population and politics. Most of these data come from government sources, and notes here direct readers to the latest updates. This chapter also includes excerpts from U.S. Supreme Court decisions and presidential rhetoric on these programs. As noted, chapter 6 includes a list of suggested further resources for those who want to learn more. Finally, the book concludes with a chronology of important developments in the history of Medicare and Medicaid and a glossary of key terms.

Acknowledgments

I remain grateful to a number of people who assisted in various ways in assembling this volume. I am particularly grateful to the contributors of chapter 3 who took their time to offer their diverse perspectives from their various perches in the complicated, fascinating, and vital world of health care: Amanda Hopkins, Adam Houghton, Tory Lynch-Dahmm, Philip Rocco, Robert Shapiro, Andrew Scholnick, and Mollie Ward. Thanks also to Madi Corey, Madison Garofalo, Clarissa King, Pooja Patil, Kayley Rettberg, and Tracy Tiritilli at Illinois Wesleyan University for their research assistance and useful feedback on the manuscript. Ann Frederick at Carle-BroMenn Medical Center lent important insights. Robin Tutt at ABC-CLIO provided invaluable guidance throughout this project.

Medicare and Medicaid

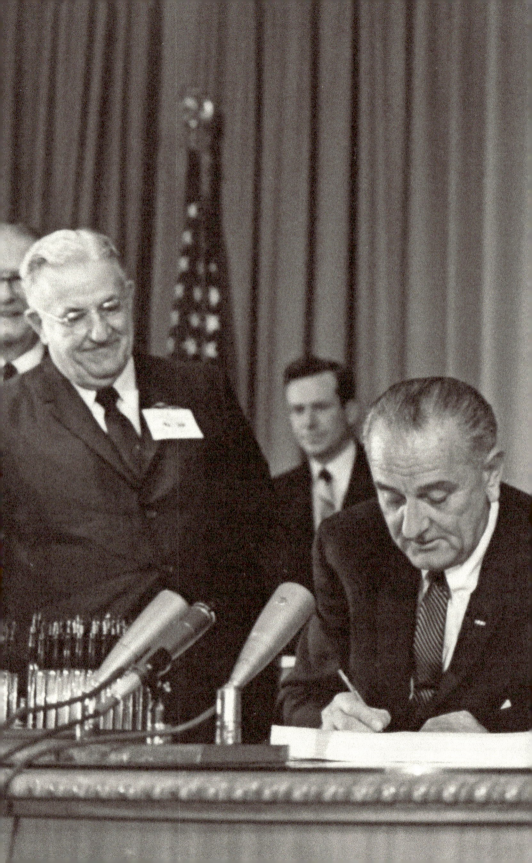

1 Background and History

The Historical Roots of Medicare and Medicaid

The history of the debate over government-provided health insurance in the United States has been defined in large part by an abiding skepticism about government involvement in the financing and delivery of services. Even after the creation of Medicare and Medicare in 1965, calls for their expansion have run into the critique that government cannot provide these services as efficiently as the private market can do. While the particulars of the arguments have changed over the decades, the skepticism that marked the early years of the debate still sound quite familiar when pronounced by contemporary advocates for or against one set of reforms or another. Even a brief telling of the history of Medicare and Medicaid makes this much clear.

The history of calls for government health insurance dates back to the 1910s. The main proposal of that era, advanced by the American Association for Labor Legislation (AALL), was to have employers, workers, and state governments share the expenses of providing for insurance. State legislatures in New York and California heard testimony on the AALL's model bill,

President Lyndon B. Johnson signs the Medicare program into law on July 30, 1965. Also present was former president Harry Truman, who became the first person to apply for the federal health care program. (Lyndon B. Johnson Library)

but the proposal failed to win passage there and was not given much consideration elsewhere. While unsuccessful as a specific bill, this campaign helped to build a community of policy advocates who would carry the general idea forward to the Franklin Roosevelt Administration. As Roosevelt's Committee on Economic Security set about drafting what would become the Social Security Act of 1935, it developed a proposal for an employment-based health insurance system that would be federally sponsored.

In the spring of 1935, out of caution President Roosevelt asked the committee to delete the health insurance language from the draft legislation for fear of the controversy derailing the larger legislative package (Altmeyer 1966; Numbers 1978). In understanding Roosevelt's fears, it is important to recall the power of opponents at the time, principally the American Medical Association (AMA), which staunchly stood against any sort of government involvement in health care. The AMA opposed even the inclusion of a modest line in the draft bill calling for federal support to study best practices in health insurance, perceiving it as too much of a threat. The administration removed the few sentences from the bill before sending it to Congress (Feingold 1966; Poen 1979). A main line of argument from the AMA was articulated by Morris Fishbein, the editor of the *Journal of the Medical Association*, who wrote in an editorial in March 1934 that the threats of socialized medicine posed by such programs would involve "hundreds of thousands of bureaucratic employees who idle through their six-hour days; they see them snooping into the intimacies of American family life, coming between the doctor and his patient, and waxing fat on the tax money extorted from wage earners and employers alike" (Burrow 1963, 203). It is important to understand that throughout the late-19th and early-20th centuries most physicians, and certainly the leadership of the AMA, saw themselves as independent businessmen, not to be interfered with by the federal or state governments. This view, combined with their frequent reference to the sacred doctor-patient relationship and to medical expertise (to the extent this can be talked about prior to the 20th century, when what we would now call medical malpractice was common), heavily drove the opposition of organized medicine to government involvement in health care provision and financing (Starr 1982).

Not all of the organized medical societies of the time consistently lined up with the AMA. The American College of Surgeons, for instance, supported a government plan to broaden health insurance. A separate group, the Committee of Physicians for the Improvement of Medicine, numbering some 400, produced in 1937 a document proposing a tax-funded national health policy. In a similar vein, and drawing an explicit contrast between his own group and the AMA, in the spring of 1938 the president of the American College of Physicians spoke out against what he called the AMA's "partisan behavior" in its opposition to a national health policy (Funigiello 2005, 31). Non-medical groups, such as the National Association for the Advance of Colored People and various farming and urban constituency organizations, testified before Congress during this period, taking the position that health care is a basic citizenship right. These arguments, however, would not carry the day, as deep skepticism persisted about government involvement in health care provision and financing for decades more.

With the support of such groups, and despite the highly organized resistance, advocacy for progressive reforms continued in Congress throughout the coming decades. Prominent in this campaign was Democratic Senator Robert Wagner of New York, who introduced a national health insurance bill in February 1939. This was the first of what would be several versions of a compulsory health insurance bill sponsored by Wagner and his Senate colleagues James Murray (Dem.) of Montana and House member John Dingell, Sr. (Dem.) of Michigan (Oberlander 2003). The bill called for the establishment of medical assistance to mothers and infants, an expansion of federal funds for the U.S. Public Health Service, increased federal funding for hospital and clinic construction, and the launch of a temporary disability payment program. All of the bill's provisions could be adopted by states voluntarily. Some reform allies, such as the Committee of Physicians for the Improvement of Medical Care, supported the bill, but the opposition both within and outside the medical community was adamant and well organized. After several months of hearings and consideration and still facing this opposition, in June 1939, Senator Murray tabled the bill (Hirshfield 1970; Funigiello 2005).

Again reacting out of caution, in late 1939 President Roosevelt shifted his support away from the Wagner-Murray-Dingell bill and opted instead to back more modest efforts to improve public health. The result turned into congressional support during the 1940s and 1950s for the less politically volatile approach of funding hospital and clinic construction. This program, enacted under the Hill-Burton Act of 1946 and derided as the "Fifty Little Hospitals Bill" by those who thought it less than ambitious, must have seemed like a blessing to the AMA and the American Hospital Association, since it provided federal financial backing for public health without any interference in the practice of medicine (Hirshfield 1970; Poen 1979).

To public health officials, medical providers, and the public, the need for more facilities was clear, especially in rural areas. The Hill-Burton Act extended federal funds to build and modernize hospitals, clinics, and nursing homes with the explicit expectation that those facilities would extend a significant amount of charity care to those unable to pay for their services. Because the grants were directed at building construction and did not directly implicate how doctors and other clinicians treated patients, this measure was relatively uncontroversial. However, problems arose in connection to the conditions attached to the grants. One important example involved a nod to racial segregationists. The Hill-Burton Act permitted segregation in places where purportedly equal facilities were available nearby. Illustrating this, North Carolina availed itself of the segregationist option under its Hill-Burton grant and constructed a pair of all-white hospitals, a pair of hospitals for Blacks, and 54 other facilities that were racially segregated by ward (Budrys 2005). Not until 1963 did the U.S. Supreme Court strike down the "separate but equal" provision. Beyond the problems of segregation, the Hill-Burton Act also favored wealthier communities and nonprofit organizations because of the dollar-for-dollar matching basis of its grants. This allowed higher resource towns and counties to draw down many more federal dollars than could poorer entities. Consequently, relatively few of the nation's poorest communities took advantage of the program (Starr 1982).

Inching closer to public funding for medical services for the indigent, in 1950 Congress created a small system of vendor payments under the Social Security amendments of that year. These payments reimbursed doctors and hospitals for treating a limited demographic group: totally and permanently disabled poor persons. This legislation marked a small but important turning point in public funding for health care provision. The majority of states welcomed the funds, and their use spread quickly. By 1960, annual federal vendor payments for the poor reached $514 million (Catlin and Cowan 2015). Though not representing a major financial commitment, this program helped set a precedent that states could administer small payments to medical providers without taking on a broad responsibility for the poor or interfering in the provision of health care to the larger population (Stevens and Stevens 1974). After a decade of experience with this program, Congress formalized the arrangement in 1960 with the passage of the Kerr-Mills program, named for Oklahoma Senator Robert Kerr and Arkansas Representative Wilbur Mills. This offered federal funds for states to reimburse medical providers who cared for poor individuals. Broadening the clientele, the Kerr-Mills program did not require beneficiaries to be disabled persons. This program, while modest in its reach, would go on to further pave the way for the 1965 adoption of Medicaid.

The growing elderly population, attributable mostly to lengthening life spans, heightened the need for medical care for senior citizens. By 1960, the typical person aged 65 or older faced a burden of medical expenses that was about twice that of the average American (Stevens and Stevens 1974). Further, seniors garnered considerable sympathy, which made it more politically palatable to extend help to this group. Elderly voters' growing share of the electorate also made them more potent politically.

For members of Congress, the enactment of the Kerr-Mills program in 1960 represented a compromise between those who wanted a universal Social Security-based system and those who fundamentally opposed federal government involvement in health care. Part of the latter's opposition stemmed from concerns about national versus state government power. The Kerr-Mills program minimized conflict by allowing states to set their own standards for financial eligibility, and it allowed states to preserve whatever administrative procedures they may have had in place earlier, including racially discriminatory ones (Stevens and Stevens 1974). Although the funding formula was designed to benefit poorer states, those that had been funding medical assistance efforts tended to be wealthier states, and this pattern continued with Kerr-Mills. While 28 of the states adopted the program by the end of 1962, only a few used it extensively. In 1965, five states (New York, California, Massachusetts, Minnesota, and Pennsylvania) accounted for 62 percent of the federal funds spent, even though these states accounted for only 31 percent of the nation's elderly population (Zelizer 2015). While the program did not challenge states to take ambitious steps to expand coverage, neither did it offend their political sensibilities. As one history on the topic put it, "The Kerr-Mills legislation rocked no boats" (Stevens and Stevens 1974, 28). Importantly, however, this assessment cuts two ways. While in the short term, the program did not lead to a broadening of access to health care by the elderly poor, it did lay the groundwork for important expansions that would occur within a few years. Because Kerr-Mills was not aggressively implemented by most states, mainly due to low reimbursement levels for providers, the percentage of senior citizens who benefited from it remained stuck in the single digits through its existence.

Despite its limitations, the Kerr-Mills program played an important role over its short life span by demonstrating that federal assistance could be blended with state efforts to cover the medical expenses of low-income seniors and that doing so would not ruin medical markets or meaningfully interfere with the doctor-patient relationship, as had been the claims of critics for decades. Hence, this program helped allay the fears associated with notions of "socialized medicine." This lesson would become crucial after the 1964 elections, which saw victories by waves of liberal supporters of government medical assistance.

The 1965 Enactment of Medicare and Medicaid

With the elections of 1964 swelling the ranks of Medicare supporters in Congress, the way for more sweeping progressive legislation rapidly opened. That year's electoral landslide gave House Democrats a more than two-to-one majority. No House candidates who supported Medicare lost in the general election. In the Senate, Democrats built slightly on their already formidable majority. This defeat for opponents forced them to recognize that some type of government-organized insurance would soon become a reality, and they responded with proposals of their own. Soon after the elections, Wilbur Mills, the chair of the House Ways and Means Committee who had stalled legislative progress for years, acknowledged that the committee would be moving forward on the King-Anderson bill, the main Democratic proposal for Medicare (Shaw 2010).

Among others who decided to come to the negotiating table, House Republicans offered what turned out to be a last-ditch effort to blunt the pent-up progressive momentum. In early 1965, Republican Representative John Byrnes offered an alternative to the King-Anderson bill. This more market-oriented approach, called Bettercare, would have coordinated voluntary insurance funded partly by premiums deducted from workers' paychecks, but not from employers themselves, and subsidized by federal government funds. The voluntary nature of this idea appealed to conservatives, but for liberals, there remained several problems. First, the Bettercare proposal allowed medical providers to assign what they thought were reasonable charges, versus set costs, which they saw as an invitation to cost overruns. Also, because Bettercare was voluntary, its reach would fall short of universalism. Further, because those enrolling would need to pay part of the premium during retirement, this would create a financial strain on seniors at a time of life when they could least afford it.

In early 1965, the American Medical Association advanced its own proposal as an alternative to the Democrats' Medicare bill. The AMA's idea, called Eldercare, proposed a voluntary plan involving a federal subsidy to private insurance purchases for seniors and an increase in federal funding for the Kerr-Mills program. The AMA remained opposed to moving away from a means test for medical assistance, since its leadership was adamant about limiting program scope (Funigiello 2005).

These three proposals—Medicare, Bettercare, and Eldercare—emerged as the major contenders under congressional consideration during the spring of 1965. Because the sponsors of these bills all sat on the Ways and Means Committee, the members of Congress were torn between competing ideas. During a committee session on March 2, the imperative to reconcile these three approaches became clear to Mills. In response, the chairman surprisingly proposed a merger of them instead of forcing a showdown. In a move that stunned many in the room, Mills asked if the committee could combine the three into one package instead of picking from among –them. This dramatic reversal has been characterized as "one of the monumental turnabouts in U.S. political history" (Steinmo and Watts 1995, 347–48). From this move emerged the famous three-layer cake metaphor: mandatory coverage for hospital services paid for by withholding payroll during one's working years, voluntary physician services paid for by monthly premiums deducted from one's Social Security payments, and a general revenue-funded program for the medically indigent. Stunning though it was, this idea enjoyed an immediate appeal among many committee members. The apparent solution also had the effect of taking the wind out of the sails of the AMA's opposition, in as much as it included their indigent care program. Further, it provided the Republicans some of what they wanted in a voluntary program, and it gave liberal Democrats the compulsory program they sought. Wilbur Cohen, Assistant Secretary of the Department of Health, Education and Welfare, noted later that "it was the most brilliant legislative move I'd seen in 30 years. The doctors couldn't complain because they had been carping about Medicare's shortcomings and about its being compulsory. And the Republicans couldn't complain, because it was their own idea" (Oberlander 2003, 30–31). The resulting bill, proposing an annual cost of just over $6 billion, reached the House floor on April 8 and was passed by a vote of 313 to 115 (Funigiello 2005).

On the Senate side, following two weeks of testimony in the Finance Committee, the bill progressed to the floor, where, after a few days of debate, it sailed through by a vote of 68 to 21 (Funigiello 2005). President Johnson signed the bill into law on July 30, 1965. Not only did this program benefit senior citizens, it benefited the Johnson Administration. A July 1964 poll found that only 14 percent of respondents thought the administration was doing a "very good" job "providing medical care for the aged." By August 1965, that figure had risen to 59 percent (polling by Opinion Research Corporation). Clearly, this was not only a substantively important achievement for the Democrats but also a popular one.

The provisions of the newly added Title XVIII of the Social Security Act, where Medicare is located statutorily, included 60 days of covered hospital care with a deductible, 30 days of hospital care beyond that with a daily co-payment, 20 days of covered nursing home care, followed by 80 more days with a daily co-payment, up to 100 home health aide visits following hospitalization, and coverage of 80 percent of the cost of diagnostic tests after a nominal deductible for each series of tests. In order to pay for the program, the taxable wage base rose to $6,600 per year, and the tax rate was increased by one-half of one percentage point for both employer and employee.

Despite the slight increases in taxation to pay for Medicare, concerns about funding would soon emerge as a serious problem. By 1967, Medicare experienced steeply escalating costs due in part to the statutory language being very permissive regarding reimbursement levels. The initial version of the act allowed the program to pay medical providers "customary, prevailing, and reasonable charges" (Oliver et al. 2004, 292). This left the door wide open for abuse and significant cost overruns. Furthermore, patients had quickly taken advantage of the services under these new programs, and providers responded with larger facilities and improved technology. Whereas medical costs had risen approximately 7 percent annually from 1950 to 1965, in the several years after 1965, hospital prices increased an average of 14 percent per year, a trend that continued into the mid-1970s (Funigiello 2005).

For federal officials, the rapidly rising costs of Medicare were shocking. To begin, the uptake rate was very strong. By the time Medicare was formally launched in July 1966, an impressive 93 percent of eligible seniors were enrolled (Marmor 1999). Within its first two years, the program had extended coverage to some 20 million people over age 65, or 10 percent of the overall population, and had paid $8.4 billion in medical bills. By early 1968, it was becoming apparent that the federal government would soon be responsible to pay for more than 20 percent of the nation's total health care expenditures. Prospective estimates generated in early 1968 estimated that this figure would reach 37 percent by 1970. The skyrocketing costs confirmed the worst fears of Medicare critics. Wilbur Mills worried out loud that Medicare was unbalancing the Social Security funding system, and he called the program one of the more serious mistakes of his career. In response to these cost increases, President Johnson urged providers to limit themselves to reasonable charges, but this effort at moral suasion appears to have had little impact (Funigiello 2005).

Rapidly rising costs catalyzed two important lines of conversation. First, efforts at cost containment gained almost immediate traction in Congress. Further, a few proponents of universal health care saw this as an opportunity to revisit calls for covering all Americans in the hopes of achieving an improved uniformity of programming and a greater economy of scale. Calls for broader government coverage would not lead to any real change, though quite a bit of effort went into cost controls, both in the states and at the federal level. A chief source of escalating costs was the statutory language permitting government reimbursements for "reasonable costs" and "customary charges" instead of specifying prices for particular services. This vagueness in the law meant the federal budget would bear whatever providers asked, and they asked for more as time passed. Complicating matters was the lack of an organizational disposition to challenge medical providers over their billing. Social Security administrators had long cultivated cooperative relationships with doctors and hospitals and planned to continue the same in the interest of smooth implementation of the new programs. Federal officials feared that aggressive efforts to limit Medicare costs would undermine this cooperation (Marmor 1999).

The new Medicaid program, located in Title XIX of the Social Security Act, created a stream of federal money to match, or even exceed, state contributions to medical assistance programs that states would administer. States were required to set financial eligibility standards, and until the 1990s, eligibility was firmly tied to those having low income. Medicaid was voluntary for states—a few delayed for years in adopting it—and for providers. Now, as then, hospitals and doctors do not have to accept Medicaid as payment, though if they do, they have to accept whatever their state program pays as full payment. That is, they cannot bill patients additionally, with the exception of specified and small co-payments. When a state adopts Medicaid, it must agree to cover at least the five core areas of service, though it may broaden that scope at its discretion. These core services include inpatient hospital care, outpatient hospital care, laboratory and X-ray services, nursing home care for persons over age 21, and physicians' services (Moore and Smith 2005/06).

Medicaid was initially made available only to children, single parents and pregnant women, the elderly poor, and the disabled. The program was not designed to move America's public insurance coverage toward universalism. True to the categorical nature of America's welfare state, several classes of people were excluded from Medicaid, including the childless and working-age adults, regardless of their income. Future expansions brought in more parents and more young people, up to age 21, but large swaths of the needy population did not enjoy any benefits from this new program. Importantly, the Medicaid legislation required states to cover nursing home care under their Medicaid programs. This newly established funding stream went on to give rise to an expanding nursing home industry during the 1960s and 1970s (Thompson 2012).

Many of the details of Medicaid policy were left to the states. However, in an aspirational gesture, Congress wrote into the law that states were to fund the program "as far as practicable under the conditions in such state" (Stevens and Stevens 1974, 57). The statute also included some more assertive features. It gave the secretary of the Department of Health, Education and Welfare the authority to withhold funds from any state not "making efforts in the direction of broadening the scope of the care and services made available under the plan and in the direction of liberalizing the eligibility requirements for medical assistance" (Stevens and Stevens 1974, 67). Depending on what one considers as good-faith efforts, Medicaid needs many years before it hit its stride as a main pillar of America's health care system. Most states soon adopted the program. The nursing home industry expanded considerably by the early 1970s. However, the program maintained its strong connection to welfare up into the 1990s, meaning millions of people who would have benefitted from it, especially the near poor, did not. This changed in most, though not all, states following the passage of the Affordable Care Act.

The enactment of Medicare and Medicaid represented a major step forward for progressive advocates. For the first time, the federal government had committed to fund health services for large swaths of the population and had done so by way of an entitlement arrangement, meaning the flow of federal dollars would be very difficult to close in the future. From another perspective, the enactment of Medicare and Medicaid represented a "useful tactical retreat" from the universalism that progressives had fought for since the 1930s (Fein 1986, 54). By settling for less and focusing on the elderly, an easy group to be sympathetic toward, this move had the effect of undercutting political support for bolder and far-reaching steps. The logic of targeting the elderly was compelling. Some three-quarters of them lacked health insurance, and approximately 35 percent of them lived below the poverty line (Fein 1986, 56). The achievement was significant, but the price paid for this compromise was high in as much as it meant a push for a more comprehensive plan would be shelved for years to come.

Challenges for Implementation

Launching two very large health care programs such as these inevitably posed administrative and other challenges for states and the federal government. However, the adoption of Medicaid by states and seniors' use of Medicare went remarkably smooth. States moved quickly to adopt Medicaid. Most states saw the new Medicaid program as a reliable, open-ended financial commitment from the federal government, one that provided more than 50 percent of the program's expenditures. Within five years, nearly all of them adopted it. Arizona was the last, in 1982. As for the seniors' ability to use Medicare, getting health providers on board was vitally important. As explained above, early on this was not a problem since the payment standards were loose to the point of the program appearing like a cash cow to vendors of medical goods and services. However, even after the reforms of the late 1960s and early 1970s that constrained payments, enrollees found their new benefit to be widely applicable. Within a decade, low-income seniors caught up with their high-income peers in terms of the frequency of doctor office visits. By doing so, they closed a gap of over 20 percent that had existed in 1964, and they showed an ability to find ample willing providers (Engel 2006; Swartz 2013).

In the way of challenges, cost overruns loomed large. Beyond this, one of the greater obstacles had to do with the continuing legacy of racial discrimination, especially by hospitals in the South. Instead of including a formal civil rights provision in the Medicare law that would have explicitly created a robust federal power to enforce non-discrimination based on race, the law instead allowed the weaker practice of asking hospitals that sought to participate to sign non-discrimination contracts. Northern Democrats believed federal administrators would interpret the law as prohibiting segregation in hospitals; thus, they declined to insist on a formal civil rights provision. This ambiguous practice also allowed Southern members of Congress to tell themselves that local facilities would to some extent be able to continue their segregationist ways. Indeed, many hospitals in the South continued to offer segregated facilities. Stubbornly refusing to cooperate, many Southern hospitals either remained outside of Medicare or wrongfully participated in the program despite their continuing discriminatory practices. Nearly another decade would pass before the endemic problem of racial discrimination under Medicare would recede into history (Marmor 1999; Kooijman 1999).

While Medicare experienced unevenness across states in the form of racial discrimination and facility use in its early years, Medicaid long has experienced tremendous cross-state differences in the range of services and reimbursement levels, based on various political and economic considerations. States establish Medicaid reimbursements, so providers' and enrollees' experiences with the program vary a great deal depending on place. Arising from this variation, and despite the federal requirement that states set their reimbursement rates high enough to attract sufficient numbers of providers to the system, somewhat limited access to providers has long posed a challenge for Medicaid enrollees in many states. A 2014 study found that 69 percent of doctors reported that they were accepting new Medicaid patients (Medicaid and CHIP Payment and Access Commission 2015). While there is no central clearinghouse for such data, there is no evidence that this figure has declined significantly in the past two decades. Poorer states face an incentive to expand their Medicaid programs because the formula for federal cost-sharing involves a sliding scale with a state's share inversely related to state per capita income. The federal share for wealthiest states is 50 percent of the cost of reimbursements to medical providers, and for the poorest, it can exceed 75 percent. Despite this incentive, in the beginning Johnson Administration officials anticipated that some states would short-change the Medicaid program. Assistant Secretary of HEW Wilbur Cohen ensured that the following paragraph was part of section 1903 of the Medicaid law:

The Secretary shall not make payments under the preceding provisions of this section to a State unless the States makes a satisfactory showing that is it is making efforts in the direction of broadening the scope of the care services made available under the plan and in the direction of liberalizing the eligibility requirements for medical assistance, with a view toward furnishing by July 1, 1975, comprehensive care and services to substantially all individuals who meet the plan's eligibility standards with respect to income and resources, including services to enable such individuals to attain or retain independence or self care. (Moore and Smith 2005/06, 50)

Cohen included this language because he was acutely aware of the historical inadequacies of state implementation of indigent medical services and wanted to push states to expand. Congress repealed this language in 1972. In broad terms, Cohen's vision has only partly been fulfilled over Medicaid's history. States have certainly expanded the eligibility and the scope of services covered over time—partly driven by federal mandates, partly on their own initiatives—but the cross-state variation in coverage was and remains dramatic. (A further discussion of this follows here and in chapter 2.)

State Medicaid Experimentation: A Departure from Freedom of Choice

Part of the cross-state variation seen in Medicaid policy has arisen thanks to waivers awarded to states by the federal government, which have allowed states to implement their programs in ways that move beyond (or violate, depending on one's point of view) the standard parameters found in Title XIX. These waiver-based innovations have significantly changed how Medicaid works and have played prominent roles in shaping the Medicaid landscape since the early 1980s. Governors and state legislators have pursued innovations ranging from financial eligibility changes to cost-sharing provisions, to work requirements, and beyond. A major area of innovation and experimentation has affected the freedom of choice that beneficiaries long have enjoyed and that traditionally allowed them to seek services from any willing provider. Such freedom of choice was made an integral part of Medicaid (and Medicare too) in 1965 as a way to assure skeptics that these programs would not interfere in patients' choice of medical providers. However, states have, especially since the 1990s, sought to save money by implementing managed care systems for their Medicaid beneficiaries. Most Medicaid beneficiaries today are enrolled in some type of managed care arrangement, and coupled with the fact that more than one-third of doctors' offices decline or restrict access by Medicaid patients, provider choice for beneficiaries is significantly limited. In the context of today's private insurance environment dominated by managed care systems, this is not unusual. However, it is important to acknowledge the sea change that this represents. Whereas public insurance skeptics once railed against what they saw as government takeovers of health care based in part on concerns about patient and provider autonomy, the prevalence of managed care systems—both public and private—has rendered this particular thread of the argument largely historic.

The catalysts for these state-level changes were twofold. The first was cost. The second had to do with changes in federal law allowing state-level experimentation. As Medicaid spending rose sharply in the 1980s (at about the same time that American health care expenditures began rising generally), state officials came to think of this program as the so-called Pac-Man of state budgets, gobbling up dollars at a ferocious rate and becoming one of the most expensive lines of programming for most states. Whereas in the late 1960s, Medicaid made up some 6 percent of the typical state's budget, by 1995 it had expanded to nearly 19 percent (Tobler and Gordon 1996), close to the 17.1 percent level where it stood in 2018.

In response, state officials pressured Congress to give them the authority to experiment with limitations on Medicaid services and to turn to managed care models. This permission came in the form of a new section, 1915c, added to Title XIX as part of the 1981 Omnibus Budget Reconciliation Act. Importantly, this new section set out procedures for states to solicit waivers to pursue home- and community-based care projects, which can be less expensive than services delivered in nursing home settings. These made a good deal of sense and were quite popular with many recipients. However, such waivers also allowed states to limit the availability of such services to specific types of beneficiaries, particular areas of their states, and to set caps on the number of such spots available (Thompson 2012). This effectively became a form of service rationing. While the Reagan Administration wanted to convert Medicaid to a block grant, a shift that would have limited the federal financial liability involved, states strongly opposed this move. However, service-limiting waivers were appealing to state officials since waivers allowed policy makers to manage costs on their own terms. By the end of the 1980s, 22 states had imposed annual limits on the number of hospital days a recipient could have, and many others limited the number of physician visits, the number of prescriptions filled per year, or the range of medicines available through the state's formulary (Katz Olson 2010). When Bill Clinton assumed the presidency, he drew on his experiences as a former governor and chair of the National Governor's Association and enthusiastically embraced the use of waivers, nearly doubling the number in effect during his presidency. By the time Congress enacted the 2005 Deficit Reduction Act, with its further grant of latitude to states to craft innovative service models, states had begun to think about ways not only to target eligibility among the elderly in need of long-term services—for example, raising the income limit to 150 percent of the federal poverty level—but also to place further limits on the types of services or recipients who could be eligible. Importantly, this allowed states to further manage their Medicaid caseloads and spending (Thompson 2012).

In an additional step toward controlling costs, many states launched attempts at remaking their Medicaid programs to be somewhat more consumer driven. These reforms include the use of personalized accounts, nominal co-payments, and telephone screening designed to minimize what critics saw as irresponsible service consumption by enrollees. One such example was West Virginia under Governor Joe Manchin in the first decade of the 2000s, which designed an elaborate series of "healthy behavior" initiatives around which the new program was structured. Healthy behaviors included attending all doctor appointments, taking prescribed medicines, and using routine checkups. Failing to adhere to these parameters resulted in beneficiaries being downgraded to the most basic Medicaid plan allowed by federal law rather than the more expansive version of the program. Further, such recipients were pushed into a managed care organization, limiting their choice of providers (Katz Olson 2010, 95–96).

These many innovations in the 1990s and early 2000s helped lay the foundations for an interesting set of maneuvers that mainly Republican-controlled states would pursue in the 2010sfollowing the enactment of the Affordable Care Act. In order to create policies that President Obama's opponents could tolerate, Republicans crafted a series of consumer-like features that the expansion population under Medicaid would have to live with, which superficially resemble private insurance. Medicaid enrollees have individual accounts attributable to them, which they must pay into in the form of monthly premiums set at very low levels, with the vast majority of the dollars coming from the state's Medicaid program. Enrollees receive monthly or quarterly statements showing the balances of these accounts. Small co-payments are required for each doctor visit. The plans reward beneficiaries financially for keeping their children's vaccinations current. These innovations give a state's Medicaid expansion the sheen of private insurance while still remaining a public program. The goal was to give these state political leaders the cover they would need to insist that what they were adopting was not Obamacare but rather a state-specific Medicaid expansion that required enrollees to experience some personal accountability—"skin in the game," as many Republicans became fond of saying—rather than simply enjoying free medical insurance at government expense (Shaw 2017).

The broader use of waivers by states to tailor their Medicaid programs is, in one regard, simply another expression of the federal-state share structure that members of Congress built into it in 1965. They imagined this to be a largely state-run low-income medical program, and although it has grown far beyond its poverty status, it still very much reflects state preferences. This has come to be critically important in the era of the Affordable Care Act and its offer of a major Medicaid expansion, discussed more in chapter 2. Beyond this, the use of waivers to make Medicaid look and feel more consumer driven, especially in Republican-controlled states, fits neatly into the framework of a larger debate about health care reform that has played out across the nation over the past couple of decades. Casting Medicaid as a privilege instead of a right, and insisting on some measure—however modest—of individual accountability, plays well politically with those who want to see that this large government program also includes elements of reciprocal obligation. Work requirements for Medicaid enrollees, for instance, represent a strong version of this philosophy. Cost sharing and other waiver-based features are also part of this same political movement. Lastly, seen in a different light, limitations on choice (such as under managed care arrangements) and access (such as under rationed services) have also helped states target their Medicaid assistance while maintaining at essentially static levels the size of the slice of the budget pie represented by this very costly program over several decades. For their part, Medicare policy makers have also been busy over the years searching for ways to limit the costs of one of the other expensive programs sponsored by the federal government. It is to this that we turn next.

Confronting Medicare Expenditures: The Prospective Payment System

Because Medicare is a very large entitlement program that makes open-ended commitments to the health costs of its beneficiaries, it has the potential to drive up budget deficits more dramatically than any other single federal program. In contrast, Social Security old-age pensions are certainly large but are limited in their amounts by federal law. Medicaid, the other member of the big three entitlements, is limited by what states are willing to spend, for federal grants to states only grow in response to specific state investments, and while those investments are large, they are limited by the states' legal inability to deficit-spend.

Given this open-ended nature of Medicare, policy makers recognized early on that program enrollees could seek services in excess, providers could provide in excess, and the rules of the program could do very little to stop profligate spending. This means, for instance, that senior citizens who might have a heightened sense of their own medical needs can frequently show up at a hospital or at a doctor's office and request a wide range of services, the provider can render that wide range of services, and Medicare has to pay for it all. From Medicare's early years to the present, a major stream of reimbursement requests has come from outpatient settings providing a wide range of diagnostic services. Since at first sight, clinicians might not be able to immediately diagnose a given patient's condition, significant batteries of examinations and lab tests might seem entirely reasonable. Inpatient settings are usually even more expensive, as they tend to treat patients with more complex problems. Overnight stays, expensive technologies, and a wide variety of services can run up bills at a rate of thousands of dollars per day. Over most of the life of Medicare, the program has paid outpatient service providers on a fee-for-service basis, meaning they are paid separately for each service they provide: every office procedure, every X-ray, every medical device, every surgery. The more services are rendered, the more a provider can bill Medicare.

With this incentive structure in mind, researchers and policy makers began work on a different way of thinking about billing in the late 1960s. They began by focusing on inpatient services. However, not until 1983 did Congress legislate the remedy that came to be called the Diagnosis Related Group (DRG) approach. Fundamentally, the DRG system seeks to standardize payments across complex mixes of patients and conditions in inpatient settings. While this prospective payment system is highly complex, the essential part to keep in mind is that Medicare places patients and their conditions into a classification system based on several factors, including the severity of their illnesses, the prognosis, the difficulty of expected treatment, the need for medical intervention to address the problems, and the intensity of resources needed. The placement of a patient into one of over 740 categories in the DRG framework determines how much a hospital will be paid to treat that particular person on that particular visit. Importantly, under this system the incentive comes to focus on efficiency rather than on volume of services. When this system was implemented in the 1980s, Medicare officials intended to force physicians and other clinicians to leave Medicare's earlier fee-for-service environment that was essentially risk-free for them and to fundamentally shift to one of efficiency and quality over quantity of services, since they would be paid a set amount determined at the beginning of the hospital admission. Over the years, there has been considerable debate among practitioners and policy makers as to how to make the list of diagnoses not only appropriately diverse and inclusive but also clinically coherent, meaning that any single patient placed in a given category will closely resemble any other patient placed in that category. Ongoing revisions to the categories have occurred, and that system was widely revised in 2007 to better account for the severity of illnesses.

Regardless of whatever quibbles that may persist over the precise design of Medicare's prospective payment system, virtually all observers agree that the DRG framework saves taxpayers a great deal of money over what Medicare would spend without it. As many actors in the private insurance market gradually shift toward bundled payments—that is, paying a set fee for a bundle of related services—this approach to a smarter payment system has become increasingly conventional across insurers. It is important to note that no such prospective payment system

exists for the Medicare outpatient domain, so clinics and doctors' offices can still enjoy a fee-for-service environment there.
This leaves a door open for very high levels of service use and
billing. For example, collectively, the top ten Medicare billing
physicians typically have filed claims for more than $100 mil-
lion each year over the past decade (Millman 2014). A minority of physicians claim that their office visits are nearly always
highly complex (this is not the norm), which nets them a larger
per-visit payment than less complex visits do (Ornstein and
Grochowski 2017). Many other high-billing physicians point
to the frequency of administering drugs that cannot be self-
administered by the patients at home. Thanks to Medicare law,
this practice earns the physician payment equal to the average
price of a dose of the drug plus 6 percent. While it is true that
most Medicare reimbursements do not cover the cost of providing the service, it is also true that many providers attempt
to overcome this problem through large-scale service billing.

Medicaid Reforms and Efforts to Control Costs

The tensions between federal and state authorities played out
in various ways during the 1980s and 1990s, as policy makers
at both levels sought to expand coverage and simultaneously to
control costs. Through this time, Congress took a series of steps
to enhance coverage for young children and pregnant women,
raising the income standards permitted for Medicaid recipients
above those normally used to establish welfare eligibility. Many
states also extended Medicaid coverage for up to six months to
families departing from the welfare rolls, which had the effect
not only of granting medical assistance to a slightly broader
population than had traditionally been eligible but was also
designed to soften the financial cliff often experienced by families departing welfare. This was not a wholesale expansion of
the program but rather an effort to target assistance to particularly vulnerable populations (Coughlin et al. 1994). These
changes can be thought of as opening moves in a long struggle

to separate Medicaid eligibility from welfare eligibility, something that would finally occur with the passage of the Affordable Care Act in 2010.

In another expansive move, Congress pushed states to pay adequate nursing home reimbursements to ensure that a critical mass of providers would remain in the Medicaid market by adopting what came to be called the Boren Amendment in 1980 (named for Senator David Boren of Oklahoma). The language of the statute called for states' payments to nursing homes to be "reasonable and adequate to meet the costs which must be incurred by efficiently and economically operated facilities in order to provide care and services in conformity with applicable state and federal laws, regulations, and quality and safety standards" (section 1902(a)(13) of the Social Security Act). This less-than-precise language led to frequent litigation, as Medicaid officials in many states saw this mandate as something that forced them to spend scarce dollars on nursing homes at the expense of other types of important services. During the Boren Amendment's first decade, providers in 29 states sued over what they saw as unreasonably low reimbursement rates. Although in 1990 the U.S. Supreme Court upheld providers' rights to bring these cases, pressure from state officials on Congress led the latter to eliminate the Boren Amendment from Medicaid law via the Balanced Budget Act of 1997 (Katz Olson 2010).

Persistently rising Medicaid costs during the 1980s led states to fight back in other ways. One was a clever scheme, referred to as bootstrapping, by which states leveraged additional federal funds through the Disproportionate Share Hospital program. This program, developed as part of the Social Security Act amendments of 1985, provides enhanced reimbursements to hospitals that serve a disproportionately high number of Medicaid enrollees. Since most Medicaid payments do not cover the costs of providing the service, to have a large share of one's patients pay with this insurance puts hospitals in a financially untenable position. As important as such augmented payment are, states quickly learned to game this system. Under this provision, many states responded with what was essentially an accounting shuffle that involved soliciting voluntary contributions from disproportionate share hospitals, placing those funds on their ledger sheet as *state* dollars dedicated to Medicaid, and consequently drawing down more federal dollars. This scheme worked for states because most states receive a matching federal payment that significantly exceeds each dollar they contribute to the program. Thus, putting in one additional dollar draws more than one dollar in federal funds. Cognizant of the overuse of this tactic, in 1991 Congress outlawed voluntary contributions from hospitals to states via the Medicaid Voluntary Contributions and Provider-Specific Tax Amendments of 1991. Always in search of more federal funds, states responded by making the assessments on their hospitals mandatory instead of voluntary; thus, this practice continues today. In a related way, states also attempted to game this system by designating more of their hospitals to be DSH facilities in order to draw down more federal funds. Congress responded by capping DSH funding to 12 percent of a state's Medicaid spending after October 1992 (Katz Olson 2010).

The Children's Health Insurance Program

One of the more consequential expansions of Medicaid in the past quarter century was the 1997 creation of the State Children's Health Insurance Program. The CHIP program is designed to provide health insurance to children whose households' income exceed the conventional standards for Medicaid but still cannot afford private health insurance. In order to be eligible, a person must be under age 19 or be the primary caretaker for a child under this age. States administer the program, including setting income standards, service scope, and administrative procedures. Typically, the program covers children living in households with income up to 200 percent of the federal poverty level ($42,660 for a family of three in 2019). States enjoy considerable flexibility with CHIP funds, allowing them to target specific types of services or even imposing deductibles and co-payments up to 5 percent of the family annual income for families with income above 150 percent of the poverty level (Katz Olson 2010).

CHIP was enacted under a Democratic president and a Republican Congress, and this political balance was reflected in the program's funding mechanism. It functions in part like an entitlement, with eligible children readily being enrolled in the program, and in part like a block grant, with dollar limits on the federal funds that are available to particular states. Funds remaining from states that do not spend their entire allotment during a given year are redistributed to other states in need, though these funds are finite (Lambrew 2007). This was not the only element of political balance built into the law. Democrats wanted to expand Medicaid for a broad swath of Americans, but they could not expect to get such a bill through a Republican-controlled Congress (though GOP support grew over the next several years). Instead, the focus on children and on state discretion proved to be a very successful formula to secure bipartisan support. Republicans have traditionally favored state leadership in matters of redistributive policy, and they got a lot of what they wanted in this compromise. Democrats wanted to see more of the vulnerable poor covered by Medicaid, and CHIP's focus on children satisfied this. In line with a long history of states showing their political preferences, states could be more or less generous, according to their liking. In the late 1990s and certainly today, the cross-state variation in financial eligibility is broad.

In the beginning, states were limited to covering children in households with income up to 250 percent of the federal poverty level. Congress, with significant bipartisan support, twice attempted to expand this during the George W. Bush Administration, though lawmakers were turned back by presidential vetoes. President Bush believed that CHIP should focus on truly low-income children and do this in a quality way rather than attempting to spread its limited resources out across families having income approaching middle class. This expansion would have enlarged the enrollment from some 6.6 million children to 10 million (Stout 2007). While Congress and President Bush could not find common ground on this, signing this expansion into law was one of President Obama's first acts in office in early 2009. Many states enthusiastically expanded their programs, with 19 states offering this assistance at or above 300 percent of the poverty level as of 2019. New York is at the high end, covering kids in households with income up to 405 percent of the poverty level (Kaiser Family Foundation 2019a).

For supporters of public health insurance, CHIP stands as a significant victory. The uninsured rate among children stood at 9.7 percent in 2008, but it dropped to 4.7 percent by 2016, largely due to the expansion of this program (Cross-Call 2018). This figure is less than half of the nation's overall uninsured rate, signaling that government efforts have had particularly good effect for the nation's children. However, this gain is far from guaranteed. In 2017, the uninsured rate among children crept up slightly to 5 percent, despite a low unemployment economy. One likely explanation is that many of the jobs added during 2017 were part-time or low-benefit, thus did not include health insurance. Compounding this, there is reason to believe that public confusion about how to access public health insurance, either through Medicaid or the online insurance exchanges, increased due to the withdrawal of government advocacy and education surrounding the ACA by the Trump Administration. Because most of the funding for health insurance exchange navigators was eliminated in 2017, many families who could have enrolled in health insurance programs did not do so (Morse 2018).

Medicare's Prescription Drug Benefit: Part D

The federal budget surpluses of the late 1990s catalyzed not only the creation of the State Children's Health Insurance Program but also a sustained conversation among policy makers about the addition of a prescription drug benefit for Medicare beneficiaries. This was an idea that had percolated in Congress since the 1960s, though concerns over the potentially very high costs had stood in the way of adoption for decades. In 1988, Congress legislated a catastrophic care module for Medicare recipients, which included a limited prescription drug benefit. However, when Congress repealed this program in 1989, because of its controversial funding mechanism (increased costs for high-income seniors), the drug benefit also ended. Not surprisingly, millions of seniors had come to appreciate the help with their medicines, and they very much missed it when it was withdrawn. Furthering the political support for prescription drug coverage under Medicare was the departure of many managed care networks in the late 1990s. Many of these plans had included some form of drug benefit. By the beginning of the new century, the stage was set for movement on this issue.

In his 1999 State of the Union Address, President Bill Clinton called for a Medicare prescription drug program, proposing a tiered arrangement with coverage based on enrollees' annual expenses: 50 percent of costs for the first $5,000 in annual spending and complete coverage of any additional costs. While Congress did not enact Clinton's plan, all of the major presidential candidates in 2000 advanced their own ideas for one. Clearly, the idea was getting some political traction. As one of the two major party nominees, Al Gore wanted to see a voluntary benefit housed within Medicare to protect the chronically ill and low-income beneficiaries. George W. Bush called for a new federal subsidy to help low-income beneficiaries purchase drugs through private insurers. Once in office, Bush proposed a block grant to states that would focus assistance on beneficiaries with incomes below 175 percent of the federal poverty level. Frustrated with the slow progress by Congress, the Bush Administration attempted to accomplish this unilaterally by executive action, but when challenged in court, the effort failed. Adding another obstacle, most beneficiaries, both

Democrats and Republicans, preferred a federally run benefit rather than a presumably weaker, state-run program such as Bush had attempted to create (Oliver et al. 2004).

Responding to the strong appetite for a benefit among the elderly, in the spring of 2002, House Republicans and Senate Democrats separately proposed outpatient drug coverage plans, though the two chambers could not agree on a single strategy at that time. When the 2002 elections gave the GOP control to both chambers, congressional leadership pushed ahead with a tiered drug plan that would become Medicare's Part D benefit. President Bush was supportive, though he indicated a strong preference that the overall cost should not exceed $400 billion over a decade. This would turn out to be a difficult threshold to maintain, both for Congress and the executive branch.

A key strategy for containing costs for a program attempting to benefit tens of millions of individuals was to define levels or tiers of coverage that varied in the coverage offered. Because of the difficulty of estimating how extensively beneficiaries would use these benefits, Congress created a three-tier system. The first tier involved an annual deductible of $250. Between this level and the initial coverage limit of $2,250, individuals would be responsible for 25 percent coinsurance (meaning the government would pay 75 percent of drug costs). For annual expenses above this initial coverage limit and up to $3,600, the plan offered no insurance at all. This was the coverage gap, or doughnut hole, put in place as an expense saver, but also in part because Congress's actuaries had difficulty generating a reliable estimate of how many enrollees would find themselves in this middle range of expenditures. However, once a person's expenses exceeded $3,600, Medicare would pay 95 percent of the costs while the beneficiary only the remaining 5 percent in what was called the catastrophic range. Over time, each of these dollar thresholds has risen. In 2019, the deductible reached $415, the initial coverage limit $3,820, and the catastrophic threshold $5,100. An enrollee's obligations vary somewhat within these tiers, as low-income individuals receive help with their enrollment fees and receive a $600 credit toward drug costs if their income is below 135 percent of the federal poverty level.

The doughnut hole has been a source of concern and consternation since its creation. Experience has shown that approximately one-quarter of beneficiaries enrolled in Medicare's Part D face drug expenses that exceed the initial coverage limit; thus, they fall into this coverage gap. Since 2014, this number has been over 10 million each year (Cubanski et al. 2018). Provisions in the Affordable Care Act have substantially narrowed this gap, lowering enrollees' obligations to only 25 percent of costs within this middle tier, matching the 25 percent coinsurance rate that applies in the tier below it.

While enrolling in Part D is not mandatory, failing to do so leads to a lifelong penalty for Medicare beneficiaries, which consists of a small increase in one's premiums. This provision is based on the same logic that Part B should be mandatory: Medicare's insurance works best when the risks are spread as broadly as possible across the population. Once seniors enroll in Part D, they select a plan they believe that best suits their medical needs. Since 2009, the average plan has involved a premium of approximately $30 per month (Cubanski et al. 2019). One's discount card is then used to purchase medicines. Part D does not involve a public option, meaning that all of these plans are administered by private insurance companies while being funded with a combination of individuals' premiums and federal tax dollars. Enrollees who have a drug benefit under a Medicare Advantage managed care plan may use this as payment rather than enrolling in Part D. These persons are not subject to the penalty for failure to enroll in Part D.

Three aspects of the congressional enactment of Medicare's Part D were particularly noteworthy. The first had to do with the inter-branch agreement that the program would not cost more than $400 billion over its first decade. In the weeks leading up to the bill's passage, the cost estimate that Congress worked with priced Part D's first decade at $395 billion, just under the $400 billion threshold that was built into Congress's budget resolution and that President Bush insisted on. Revising the analysis, Richard Foster, Medicare's chief actuary, concluded in the summer of 2003 that the new program was more likely to cost $534 billion (Aaron and Lambrew 2008, 8). However, Foster was directed by the administrator for the Center for Medicare and Medicaid Services, the agency that operates these programs, not to release this revised cost estimate, with the threat that Foster would be fired from his job if he did. The higher figure only became public knowledge in January 2004, almost two months after the bill's passage. Had this much higher estimate seen the light of day earlier, one of two outcomes would have been quite likely. First, the bill probably would not have survived the opposition of fiscal conservatives in Congress. Alternatively, members would have built in cost controls on drugs, a move strongly opposed by the pharmaceutical industry (PhRMA no date). In the end, cost controls were not built into Part D. Looking back, Medicare's Part D annual expenditures rose from about $46 billion in 2007 to $80 billion in 2017, growing at an annual rate of 5.7 percent over that decade (Medicare Payment Advisory Commission 2019). This level of spending turned out to be less than initially expected, due mainly to lower price inflation among drugs and because fewer Medicare recipients have enrolled in Part D than projected back in the early 2000s (Congressional Budget Office 2014; Hoadley et al. 2015).

The absence of cost controls leads to a second curious turn in the legislative process. It was perhaps unexpected that Medicare's Part D would be finally moved across the legislative finish line by Republicans rather than Democrats, given the historical partisan alignments on issues regarding America's welfare state. One particular provision in the Medicare Modernization Act of 2003 particularly defies conventional thinking about what constitutes political conservatism and how free markets ought to be regarded while making public policy.

During the final stages of negotiations over Part D, many conservative Republicans expressed qualms about the large expense of this package and the expansion of Medicare more generally. Republican leaders in the House of Representatives were particularly concerned that they would not secure enough votes to clear the measure for the president's signature. (Twenty-five House Republicans ultimately voted against the measure.) In an unusual parliamentary move, Speaker Dennis Hastert, a sponsor of the bill, extended floor voting for three hours (beyond its typical 15 minutes), during which GOP leaders pressured several members to switch their votes from "no" to "yes." At least one Republican member later commented that he had been not only pressured but also offered a bribe to change his vote (Aaron and Lambrew 2008). Of key importance, Republican members needed reassurance that the government would not overly involve itself in the pharmaceutical market, so the "noninterference clause" was added to section 8060 D-11 of the bill that prohibits the Secretary of Health and Human Services from using Medicare's bulk purchasing power to negotiate lower prices (Oliver et al. 2004; Pear and Toner 2003). Supporters of this provision argue that government should not interfere in negotiations between drug makers and Medicare-managed care insurers and that to allow government involvement would lead to the government setting the prices. They further argue that this could lead to government dictating which drugs Medicare would pay for. Opponents point out that it is unreasonable that drug makers can act in profit-seeking ways while the Medicare program, by far the largest single customer, is outlawed from acting like a savvy shopper. Even though this stands in opposition to four other federal entities that are permitted to negotiate lower drug prices—the Veteran's Administration, the Department of Defense, the Public Health Service, and the Coast Guard—this arrangement carried the day in 2003 and has persisted since then. In the end, the Medicare Modernization Act was passed by the House by 216 to 215 votes (Lopert and Moon 2007; Oliver et al. 2004).

Finally, all persons who are simultaneously eligible for Medicare and Medicaid (for instance, both poor and elderly) now receive their prescription benefits through Medicare, meaning the federal government has assumed the majority of the obligation for these dual eligible individuals. To help balance the burden, states must make payments to Medicare, which approximate the savings their Medicaid programs experienced under this law. However, the formula for these state payments is such that states pay only a small amount, 10 percent on average in 2015 (Aaron and Lambrew 2008). The White House initially had concerns about the federal assumption of this funding, thinking of it as an undue financial windfall for state governments (Blum 2006, 2). For its part, the pharmaceutical industry favored the shift of dual eligibles, since it would involve a single Medicare formulary, or a list of covered drugs, instead of numerous state-specific formularies. Whatever the reasons, this shift of obligation for drugs from states to the federal government was of major consequence, especially given the steeply rising costs of many drugs over recent years.

The addition of the prescription drug benefit to Medicare is easily one of the most significant expansions of America's social insurance framework since the creation of Medicare and Medicaid in 1965. In 2018, Part D accounted for nearly one out of every five Medicare dollars spent, and the Medicare Trustees project that drug spending will continue to increase faster than other medical spending in the coming years (Kaiser Family Foundation 2019b). This assistance has obviously been a boon not only for recipients but also for the drug industry. As more lifesaving drugs come on the market, this is clearly a net positive for America's senior citizens, but as drug prices continue to rise faster than does the country's wealth, taxpayers will increasingly feel a growing burden.

Medicare and Managed Care: Part C

Just as managed care systems have expanded in the domain of private health insurance, they have also spread greatly for

Medicare recipients. By 2018, fully 45 percent of Medicare enrollees were part of a managed care plan (Jacobson et al. 2018). The primary attraction for enrollees to sign up is the minimization of the many co-payments and deductibles that traditional Medicare involves. In exchange, seniors who elect to enroll in one of the many privately administered managed care plans offered to them agree to limit the range of medical providers and in some cases services that would otherwise be available. This limitation likely is the dominant explanation for why Medicare managed care enrollees tend to be healthier overall than those enrolled in traditional Medicare, which involves few of such limits (McGuire et al. 2011).

Not only have nearly one-half of seniors on Medicare embraced managed care arrangements, but also members of Congress did as well when they began to create this framework in the early 1970s. The expectation was that this would help deliver good-quality medicine at lower cost—thanks to the bundling of patients into service groups—than would the traditional fee-for-service payment system. What is now called Medicare Advantage, or Part C, traces its roots to the 1972 Social Security Act amendments. That legislation created the health maintenance organization (or HMO) enrollment and contracting abilities for Medicare. Congress built on this by passing the HMO Act in 1973. In general terms, this allowed private insurers to offer capitated, or per person, plans open to all interested Medicare beneficiaries in a given service area. Regulations were finalized, and the first demonstration projects began in 1976 (McGuire et al. 2011). As is turns out, very few HMOs took up Medicare on the offer. By 1979, there were only 32 group practice payment plans, 32 HMO cost contractors, and only 1 risk-sharing HMO (Zarabozo 2000).

Responding to this very modest update, Congress enacted the Tax Equity and Fiscal Responsibility Act (TEFRA) in 1982. This allowed private insurers to receive prospective capitated payments for Medicaid enrollees in exchange for assuming full risk for their health care costs. The administrative regulations for TEFRA were finally prepared by 1985, but the incentives in the market were not yet powerful enough to cause Medicare managed care to blossom at that time. The turning point would come in the mid-1990s when insurers had worked out their business models for managed care (on the private side first, then translated it to Medicare); rising costs overall gave them stronger incentives to get it right, and the failure of the Clinton plan made it evident that it would be up to insurers to tackle the increasingly steep health spending cost curve. The name of this program began as Medicare + Choice, and it later became commonly referred to as Medicare Part C, or Medicare Advantage.

Despite being quite popular among enrollees, Medicare Advantage has not generated the expected savings for the U.S. Treasury, and this has become a sore point for many members of Congress (McGuire et al. 2011). At its most basic level, Medicare managed care arrangements are attractive to private insurers because of the ability to share in the savings they potentially generate. If a managed care plan can deliver quality services at a per capita cost that is lower than the average per capita cost for traditional Medicare enrollees in the same county, the managed care organization shares in the savings, with the federal government accruing the balance. As various observers have noted, there seems to be a fundamental conflict between the two main goals of Medicare managed care. As McGuire and colleagues write, "Medicare has not been able to find payment rules that simultaneously expand beneficiaries' choice *and* save Medicare program funds" (McGuire et al. 2011, 292). By the early 1990s, it became apparent that Part C per capita costs were approximately 6 percent higher for per capita costs for traditional Medicare (Gage 1998). Part of the problem is that the capitation rates being paid to the HMOs are not quite fine-tuned enough. Medicare enrollees who sign up for Part C tend to be healthier than those in the traditional plan (likely because intensive users, the sick, know that they would not like being restricted by an HMO, thus they stay in the traditional pool).

This means that Medicare is paying the managed care plans on a per capita basis set in reference to a less-healthy, more service-intensive traditional Medicare population.

For their part, of course, enrollees don't need to care about the inefficiencies in the system. They know that as individuals they like the services. Medicare HMO enrollment doubled from 1993 to 1999, reaching 81 million (Zarabozo 2000). Naturally, it would be politically difficult to trim these benefits, now that some 20 million seniors have grown to enjoy their enhanced coverage. As of 2009, this expansion of beneficiary choice has cost Medicare an estimated 114 percent of what traditional Medicare costs, or $14 billion extra (Patel and Guterman 2017). The passage of the Affordable Care Act has slightly trimmed Medicare Advantage's costs, as payments were frozen for 2011 and reduced slightly during 2012 and 2013. However, this temporary freeze of reimbursements does not constitute a long-term solution for what is apparently a more fundamental problem.

Medicaid Expansion under the Affordable Care Act

The most recent major development in Medicaid has been the expansion option offered to states under the Affordable Care Act of 2010. This option was available for states beginning in 2014 and allows states to cover individuals in families with income up to 138 percent of the federal poverty level. At the outset, the federal government paid 100 percent of the costs associated with the expansion population, a figure that tapered to 90 percent by 2020 (Snyder and Rudowitz 2015). Despite this very generous offer from Congress, most GOP-controlled states declined it initially, citing their unwillingness to cooperate with what they saw as an inappropriate exercise of federal authority (Shaw 2017; Béland et al. 2016). Beginning in late 2014, some of these Republican-controlled states found ways to overcome the politics and buy into the expansion, given that to not do so would leave many millions of federal dollars unclaimed. While not all of the states have taken up this initiative, as of the summer of 2019, fully 36 states and the District of Columbia had (Kaiser Family Foundation 2019a). This expansion and the political debates surrounding it raise many vital questions for public health, family and state budgets, and the well-being of medical providers.

The decision by congressional Democrats to expand Medicaid to cover the near-poor was part of a larger effort to drive down the percentage of Americans without health insurance. As John McDonough, a lead staff member for the late Senator Edward Kennedy, explained it, the threshold of 135 percent seemed to the lawmakers as a level that they could get through the Senate. This was not based on any real analysis about its consequences for public health. They also thought that because Congress would pay the vast majority of the expansion costs the states would readily accept it. In this assumption, they fundamentally miscalculated the depth of Republican resistance and the vitriol directed toward Obamacare and what it would mean to be seen as cooperating with what many of them characterized as a Washington takeover of health care. When multiple states and other organizations challenged the expansion in federal court, the states ultimately prevailed. As the Supreme Court ruled in 2012 in *National Federation of Independent Businesses v. Kathleen Sebelius*, when Congress made the expansion mandatory it had abused the fine balance of American federalism. The Court ruled that non-cooperating states could not be sanctioned by the federal government; thus, the ruling effectively made the expansion voluntary.

The result was a nearly perfect partisan alignment, with Democratic states adopting the expansion during 2014, its first year, and nearly all Republican states rejecting it. The arguments on the Republican side ranged from concerns about whether Congress would keep its promise and continue to fund the expansion population to ideological concerns about expanding another part of the American welfare state, to claims of already tight state budgets. However strident these critiques, starting in late 2014, a handful of Republican states began seeking ways to expand by crafting expansion programs that conveyed local design and ownership—the "Healthy Michigan" and "Healthy Indiana" plans were typical of this nomenclature—and that involved features of individual accountability for looking after one's health (Altman 2014). A much-copied model carried nominal monthly premiums, co-payments for office visits, and rewards for keeping up on preventative services. In several states, this veneer of individual accountability gave Republican governors and legislators the political cover they needed to adopt the Medicaid expansion (Shaw 2017).

Of course, some states have been so staunchly opposed that they have not moved in this direction. Texas is the largest population example. By not expanding Medicaid Texas, left some 759,000 persons uninsured, as of 2017, who otherwise would be covered. Nationally, this figure was approximately 2.5 million, the vast majority of them Southerners. Across the expansion states, as of 2017, just over 17 million more people had gained health insurance (Garfield et al. 2019).

An important catalyst for state adoption of the Medicaid expansion has been pressure from medical providers. Although Medicaid typically reimburses providers at much lower levels than does private insurance, nearly all hospitals and most doctors view a low reimbursement to be better than no reimbursement, which is what they receive if a patient cannot pay the bill. Because uncompensated care at the nation's 5,262 hospitals amounted to $38.4 billion in 2017, this is obviously a major concern, and the decision to support the Medicaid expansion seems like a reasonable one (American Hospital Association 2019).

The political arguments over using Medicaid to cover more Americans will almost certainly persist for years to come, likely until some type of universal coverage is devised. As a program that has, since its inception, depended on state cooperation, this major pillar of the health care system will continue to display considerable cross-state variation, and Americans' consistent access to care will continue to be in large part a function of the states in which they live.

Looking Back, Looking Forward

While history is not deterministic of future outcomes, it can certainly exert powerful influences. Decisions made a half century ago when Medicare and Medicaid were created still resonate in the way the programs work, who they benefit, funding sources, and the political debates surrounding them. Medicare's financing still draws on the same mix of sources as it always has: a combination of payroll taxes, general revenues, and individual premiums. Medicare still focuses as it always has on the elderly and is available regardless of income. Medicaid is still limited to low-income Americans. States still administer 50 Medicaid programs, and they vary in ways that reflect state-level political preferences and financial resources. Although Congress has severed the historic link between Medicaid and welfare eligibility, the means tests that screen out most Americans still prevail. Both programs bear the imprints of moments when national lawmakers were persuaded about the neediness and deservingness of vulnerable groups, whether that was the elderly or poor single parents and their children.

But the passage of five decades, the evolution of medical technology, and changing demographics and social norms have also wrought large changes in both of these programs. What started out as a welfare medicine program for single parents and their children has grown into a program that spends most of its funds on nursing homes and other long-term care, mainly for the elderly. On the Medicare side, what started out as a program that assiduously avoided influencing how doctors and hospitals practice medicine has come to shape these clinical practices through limits on payments and pressures to meet quality standards. Recent calls for some version of Medicare for All face a series of daunting obstacles, including financial, ideological, and administrative. While sweeping policies occasionally occur—consider the passage of the Social Security Act in 1935 and Medicare and Medicaid's creation in 1965—these happen only infrequently.

This chapter has focused on the key moments in the history of these two programs and developments that are most relevant to current debates. Despite progress discussed here, there persist many problems and controversies. Chapter 2 addresses some of the most important ones, along with potential solutions.

Sources

Aaron, Henry, and Jeanne Lambrew. 2008. *Reforming Medicare: Options, Tradeoffs, and Opportunities.* Washington, D.C.: Brookings Institution Press.

Altman, Drew. 2014. "Medicaid Expansion in Red States," report from the Kaiser Family Foundation (December 18).

Altmeyer, Arthur. 1966. *The Formative Years of Social Security.* Madison: The University of Wisconsin Press.

American Hospital Association. 2019. "Uncompensated Hospital Care Cost Fact Sheet" (January).

Béland, Daniel, Philip Rocco, and Alex Wadden. 2016. *The Obamacare Wars: Federalism, State Politics, and the Affordable Care Act.* Lawrence: University Press of Kansas.

Blum, Jonathan. 2006. "A History of Creating the Medicare Prescription Drug Benefit," a report from Avalere Health (August).

Budrys, Grace. 2005. *Our Unsystematic Health Care System, 2nd edition.* New York: Rowman & Littlefield Publishers, Inc.

Burrow, James. 1963. *AMA: Voice of American Medicine.* Baltimore: The Johns Hopkins University Press.

Catlin, Aaron, and Cathy Cowan. 2015. "History of Health Spending in the United States, 1960–2013," report from the Centers for Medicare and Medicaid Services, Washington, D.C. (November 19).

Congressional Budget Office. 2014. "Competition and the Cost of Medicare's Prescription Drug Program," Washington, D.C. (July).

Coughlin, Teresa, Leighton Ku, and John Holanhan. 1994. *Medicaid since 1980: Costs, Coverage, and the Shifting Alliance between the Federal Government and the States.* Washington, D.C.: The Urban Institute Press.

Cross-Call, Jesse. 2018. "Children's Uninsured Rate Rises for First Time in a Decade," report from the Center for Budget and Policy Priorities, Washington, D.C. (November 30).

Cubanski, Juliette, Anthony Damico, and Tricia Neuman. 2019. "10 Things to Know About Medicare Part D Coverage and Costs in 2019," report by the Kaiser Family Foundation (June 4).

Cubanski, Juliette, Tricia Neuman, and Anthony Damico. 2018. "Closing the Medicare Part D Coverage Gap: Trends, Recent Changes, and What's Ahead," report from the Kaiser Family Foundation (August 21).

Engel, Jonathan. 2006. *Poor People's Medicine: Medicaid and American Charity Care since 1965.* Durham, NC: Duke University Press.

Fein, Rashi. 1986. *Medical Care, Medical Costs.* Cambridge, MA: Harvard University Press.

Feingold, Eugene. 1966. *Medicare: Policy and Politics, A Case Study and Policy Analysis.* San Francisco: Chandler Publishing Company.

Funigiello, Philip. 2005. *Chronic Politics: Health Care Security from FDR to George W. Bush.* Lawrence: University of Kansas Press.

Gage, Barbara. 1998. "The History and Growth of Medicare Managed Care." *Generations* 22 (2): 11–18.

Garfield, Rachel, Kendal Orgera, and Anthony Damico. 2019. "The Coverage Gap: Uninsured Poor Adults in States That Do Not Expand Medicaid," report from the Kaiser Family Foundation (March 21).

Hirshfield, Daniel. 1970. *The Lost Reform: The Campaign for Compulsory Health Insurance in the United States from 1932 to 1943*. Cambridge, MA: Harvard University Press.

Hoadley, Jack, Juliette Cubanski, and Patricia Neuman. 2015. "Medicare Part D at Ten Years: The 2015 Marketplace and Key Trends, 2006–2015," report from the Kaiser Family Foundation (October 5).

Jacobson, Gretchen, Anthony Damico, and Tricia Neuman. 2018. "A Dozen Facts about Medicare Advantage," report from the Kaiser Family Foundation (November).

Kaiser Family Foundation. 2019a. "March 2019 Fact Sheet."

Kaiser Family Foundation. 2019b. "10 Essential Facts About Medicare and Prescription Drug Spending" (January 19).

Katz Olson, Laura. 2010. *The Politics of Medicaid*. New York: Columbia University Press.

Kooijman, Jaap. 1999. *And the Pursuit of National Health: The Incremental Strategy toward National Health Insurance in the United States*. Atlanta, GA: Rodopi.

Lambrew, Jeanne. 2007. "The State Children's Health Insurance Program: Past, Present, and Future," report from the Commonwealth Fund (February 1).

Lopert, Ruth, and Marilyn Moon. 2007. "Toward a Rational, Value-Based Drug Benefit for Medicare." *Health Affairs* 26 (6): 1,666–73.

Marmor, Theodore. 1999. *The Politics of Medicare, 2nd edition*. New York: Aldine de Gruyter Publishing Co.

McGuire, Thomas, Joseph Newhouse, and Anna Sinaiko. 2011. "An Economic History of Medicare Part C." *The Milbank Quarterly* 89 (2): 289–332.

Medicaid and CHIP Payment and Access Commission. 2015. "An Update on the Medicaid Primary Care Payment Increase," Washington, D.C. (March).

Medicare Payment Advisory Commission. 2019. "Report to the Congress: Medicare Payment Policy," Washington, D.C. (March).

Millman, Jason. 2014. "The Top 10 Medicare Billers Explain Why They Charged $121M in One Year," *The Washington Post* (April 9).

Moore, Judith, and David Smith. 2005/06. "Legislating Medicaid: Considering Medicaid and Its Origins." *Health Care Financing Review* 27 (2): 4552.

Morse, Susan. 2018. "CMS Cuts Affordable Care Act Navigator Funding from $36 to $10 Million," report from *Healthcare Finance* (July 11).

Numbers, Ronald. 1978. *Almost Persuaded: American Physicians and Compulsory Health Insurance, 1912–1920*. Baltimore: Johns Hopkins University Press.

Oberlander, Jonathan. 2003. *The Political Life of Medicare*. Chicago: University of Chicago Press.

Oliver, Thomas, Philip Lee, and Helene Lipton. 2004. "A Political History of Medicare and Prescription Drug Coverage." *The Milbank Quarterly* 82 (2): 283–354.

Ornstein, Charles, and Ryann Grochowski. 2017. "Some Doctors Still Billing Medicare for the Most Complicated, Expensive Office Visits," report from ProPublica (December 27).

Patel, Yash, and Stuart Guterman. 2017. "The Evolution of Private Plans in Medicare," report from the Commonwealth Fund (December 8).

Pear, Robert, and Robin Toner. 2003. "G.O.P. Begins Push for Medicare Bill," *The New York Times* (November 17).

PhRMA. n.d. Website discussion of Medicare Part D. Available at www.phrma.org/en/Advocacy/Medicare/PartD (accessed October 22, 2019).

Poen, Monte. 1979. *Harry S. Truman versus the Medical Lobby*. Columbia: University of Missouri Press.

Shaw, Greg M. 2010. *The Healthcare Debate*. Santa Barbara, CA: Greenwood Press.

Shaw, Greg M. 2017. *The Dysfunctional Politics of the Affordable Care Act*. Santa Barbara, CA: Praeger Publishers.

Snyder, Laura, and Robin Rudowitz. 2015. "Medicaid Financing: How Does It Work, and What Are the Implications," report from the Kaiser Family Foundation (May 20).

Starr, Paul. 1982. *The Social Transformation of American Medicine: The Rise of a Sovereign Profession and the Making of a Vast Industry*. New York: Basic Books.

Steinmo, Sven, and Jon Watts. 1995. "It's the Institutions, Stupid! Why Comprehensive National Health Insurance Always Fails in America." *Journal of Health Politics, Policy and Law* 20 (2): 329–72.

Stevens, Robert, and Rosemary Stevens. 1974. *Welfare Medicine in America: A Case Study in Medicaid*. New York: Macmillan.

Stout, David. 2007. "Bush Vetoes Children's Health Bill," *The New York Times* (October 3).

Swartz, Katherine. 2013. "Medicare and Medicaid," in Martha Bailey and Sheldon Danzinger (eds.), *Legacies of the War on Poverty*. New York: Russell Sage Foundation.

Thompson, Frank. 2012. *Medicaid Politics: Federalism, Policy Durability, and Health Reform*. Washington, D.C.: Georgetown University Press.

Tobler, Laura, and Dianna Gordon. 1996. "Will Managed Care Be Jekyll or Hyde for States?" *State Legislatures* 22 (April): 59–65.

Zarabozo, Carlos. 2000. "Milestone in Medicare Managed Care." *Health Care Financing Review* 22 (1): 61–67.

Zelizer, Julian. 2015. "The Contentious Origins of Medicare and Medicaid," in Alan Cohen, David Colby, Keith Wailoo, and Julian Zeliser (eds.), *Medicare and Medicaid at 50: America's Entitlement Programs in the Age of the Affordable Care Act*. New York: Oxford University Press.

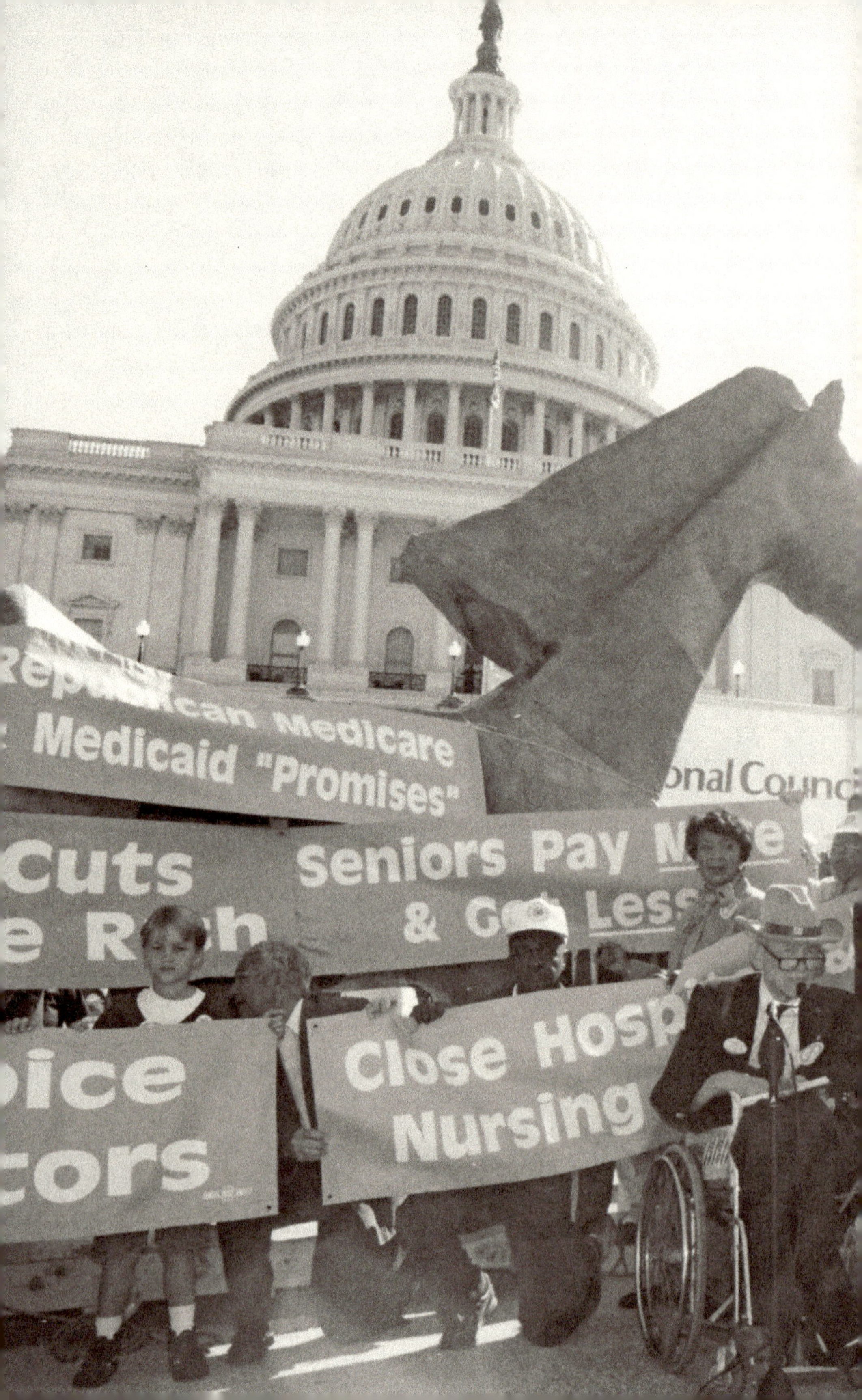
Medicaid "Promises"
Cuts
Seniors Pay
Close Hosp
Nursing
onal Counc

2 Problems, Controversies, and Solutions

The complexity of the Medicare and Medicaid programs means that the number of stakeholders for these programs is vast, reform efforts are politically complicated, and the expenses great. This chapter explains eight current policy problems or challenges. Several of these issues arise from unresolved debates that have raged for years and that were highlighted in Chapter 1. Others are the results of recent developments. For each problem, readers will find a description of the challenges, an explanation of how the issue matters for current politics and the well-being of beneficiaries or potential beneficiaries, and some discussion of proposed or attempted solutions where these apply. Many of the advocates profiled in Chapter 4 play important roles here.

The first challenge identified here is Medicare's high cost. This broad issue affects many of the others discussed in this book. Beyond describing some of the reasons that Medicare costs so much, the discussion turns to distinct options to respond to this situation. These include three very different directions. First, some advocates resist calls for program expansion and argue that policy makers should protect the program's status quo. Second, other advocates say that Congress should

A Medicare/Medicaid rally in front of U.S. Capitol, showing protesters holding signs around a "trojan horse" figure representing the Democrats' interpretation of the Republican Medicare plan, on September 29, 1995. (Library of Congress)

effectively expand Medicare by adopting a public insurance option. Third, others hope to achieve program savings through the adoption of a premium-support model, which would limit annual expenditures while placing an enlarged financial responsibility on enrollees as they shop for private insurance plans that would be subsidized by fixed government payments. The second and third options would involve significant legislation that would be highly controversial, thus resisted by well-organized stakeholders.

Problem #1: Medicare's Spending Is High and Not Well Controlled

Placing Medicare's very large expenditures in context can be a fraught exercise. As one of the most expensive lines of programming sponsored by the federal government, it represents not only a strong statement of what members of Congress and their constituents value but also speaks to what the national treasury can support. Currently, Medicare expenditures are exceeded only by outlays for Social Security and national defense. Complaints that the government spends too much on Medicare are usually predicated on the belief that health care for seniors and the disabled should be a lower public-sector priority than it currently is and that individuals should bear more of the financial burden themselves. This argument about priorities is not one to be settled here. However, it is important to consider the facts about Medicare's cost and to place these costs in the context of the overall federal budget, as a portion of the gross domestic product, and in terms of the efficiency and effectiveness of the program.

Based on the 2019 report of the Medicare Trustees, the official auditors of the program, annual Medicare expenditures amounted to 3.7 percent of the U.S. gross domestic product in 2016. Under current law, this figure is projected to rise to 4 percent by 2022 and to 6 percent by 2043, due mostly to rising per capita expenditures on the program. This growing share of the nation's resources will, of course, also be dramatically reflected in the share of the overall federal budget spent on Medicare. As of 2019, Medicare consumed 15 percent of the federal budget. By 2028, this share is expected to reach 18 percent (Cubanski and Neuman 2018). Looking at it differently, it is important to bear in mind that Medicare is the largest single health care payer in the United States today and that it funds about four of every 10 hospitals stays. Indisputably, Medicare is a key part of the American health care landscape. Framing the cost this way poses the question of how much of a priority the program should be and how willing Americans are to trim spending on many other projects, whether those are education, the environment, the Defense Department, highways, or any number of other areas. If there is good news here, it is that the Trustees' 75-year projection anticipates Medicare spending to remain nearly stable at approximately 6 percent of GDP through the foreseeable future. Taking the long view, however, also highlights the unfunded liability built into Medicare's future. The Trustees anticipate that, over the coming 75 years, the gap between promised benefits and projected revenue will range between $28 trillion and $37 trillion, depending on the actuarial assumptions used (Medicare Trustees 2019).

In understanding Medicare's cost trajectory, one must keep in mind that total expenditures through time have risen somewhat as a function of growing enrollment but even more so in terms of per capita spending. For instance, from 1975 to 2007 the percentage of the U.S. population on Medicare rose by 25 percent (from 12 to 15), but the overall expenditures more than doubled (Aaron and Lambrew 2008). Much of this per capita increase is due to advancing technology and rising demand for complicated and expensive treatments. Another portion of the increase is attributable to rising prescription drug prices. Both of these trends are also associated with an aging population. On average, seniors in their 70s consume more services than do those in their 60s. Of course, rising enrollment is also consequential, as this will force Medicare's financing and the politics surrounding that into the forefront of national debates about budgets and governmental responsibility. As of 2018, 16 percent of Americans were 65 years or older. As the population continues to age, this percentage is projected to reach 19.3 by 2030 and 20.2 by 2050 (Census Bureau 2018). The strains this will place on old-age programs generally and Medicare in particular will become a key political challenge for national policy makers. Accentuating this, the portion of senior citizens who are 75 or more years old will continue to grow through the early 2040s. Given this, the problems of funding Medicare will worsen for the next two decades before leveling out.

Of Medicare's two trust funds, the Hospital Insurance Fund (Part A), which pays for inpatient services, poses a particular challenge. The HI Fund relies heavily on payroll taxes for its revenue, typically about 85 percent. Because the tax rate is set by Congress (currently 1.45% for most workers and the same percentage for their employers) and is politically more difficult to adjust, this has put the HI Fund on a deficit trajectory. The Medicare Trustees expect it to be unable to meet its full obligations starting in 2026. At that point, Congress will have to decide to increase the payroll tax rate, or institute benefit reductions, or agree to use general revenue to bridge the gap (Medicare Trustees 2019).

Medicare's other trust fund, the Supplemental Medical Insurance Fund, covers outpatient services, or Part B. Approximately three-quarters of its funding comes from general revenue, with monthly premiums paid by beneficiaries making up nearly all of the remainder. Because the premium automatically increases each year in line with inflation, and because by law this part of Medicare has ready access to general revenue funds, the SMI Trust Fund is projected to be able to meet its obligations for the foreseeable future. While most of the discussion in this chapter will treat Medicare expenditures as though they come from a single source, readers should be aware that Congress must, by law, attend to these important accounting distinctions.

Beyond questions about how taxpayers are expected to fund Medicare, there has been much debate about the program's efficiency. Several points of reference support the idea that Medicare delivers a great deal of value for the money spent, as compared to most private health insurance policies. Such evidence has helped catalyze calls to expand Medicare to cover more of the non-elderly population, such as the Medicare for All discussions that have been prominent since about 2016. Whether a majority of Americans want to move in this direction is, of course, a matter for elections to settle.

Medicare's efficiency largely stems from its modest reimbursement rates to providers. Depending on the particular analysis and moment in time, Medicare pays between 50 and 75 percent of what the average private health insurance policy would pay for a given service, though there is substantial variation on this across place and service (Congressional Budget Office 2017). A 2017 analysis by the American Hospital Association found that, on average, Medicare pays only 87 cents for every dollar hospitals actually spend on beneficiaries' care, creating a gap of $53.9 billion that year (American Hospital Association 2019). Despite this pattern of paying less, the vast majority of providers remain in the Medicare market because they see a low payment to be better than no payment, which is what many patients would offer if not for their government insurance. While to accept Medicare as payment is voluntary for doctors and hospitals, they strongly tend to accept such customers. Surveys over the past decade have found that most doctors' offices were willing to accept new Medicare patients at a rate only slightly lower than they were willing to take on new private-pay patients (Holgash and Heberlein 2019). The story is different on the Medicaid side. See more in the following.

The lower payment rates typically translate to a loss for providers. According to the Medicare Payment Advisory Commission (MedPAC), Congress's main information agency on these matters, in 2017 hospitals on average operated at a 9.9 percent loss with their Medicare patients. Even the country's

291 most efficient hospitals (defined by MedPAC staff) experienced on average a 2.2 percent loss on Medicare patients that year (Medicare Payment Advisory Commission 2018). Clearly, even with operation-enhancing improvements, breaking even with Medicare patients is and will continue to be quite difficult. Attending to this problem has become a key goal for most hospital administrators because, for typical hospitals, between one-third and one-half of their revenue comes from Medicare patients. This heavy Medicare dependence has driven lively conversations among business consultants in the health sector about how to get to the breakeven point. This pursuit has been complicated over the past decade, as Medicare reimbursement rates have fallen somewhat under the Affordable Care Act. Of course, this also serves as a reality check for advocates who want to expand Medicare significantly beyond the population it presently serves. Medicare for All would be not only a significant shift for taxpayers, but it would also require sweeping operational changes on the part of medical providers.

One other area of controversy regarding Medicare's spending has to do with overhead administrative expenses. As it turns out, Medicare's administrative costs are substantially lower than those of private insurers. According to a 2011 analysis by the Kaiser Family Foundation, Medicare operating expenses average around 2 percent of total expenditures (Potetz et al. 2011). The average private insurer, in sharp contrast, spends approximately 20 percent of its gross revenue on administrative costs and profits (Papanicolas et al. 2018). This target was explicitly recognized in the writing of the Affordable Care Act. One of the ACA's provisions, referred to as the medical loss ratio requirement, penalizes private insurers if they fail to spend at least 80 percent of their revenues paying claims to improve the health of individuals and small groups, instead of administrative overhead, salaries, and marketing. This requirement is 85 percent for large groups of customers. Many health insurers struggle to meet this requirement (Woolhandler and Himmelstiein 2017).

Attempting to improve Medicare's efficiency further, Congress has directed the Centers for Medicare and Medicaid Services, the agency within the U.S. Department of Health and Human Services that administers this, to strengthen clinical data registries to gather information that clinicians can use to track their performance and enhance their effectiveness and efficiency. This framework was made more robust as part of the 2012 American Taxpayer Relief Act (Government Accountability Office 2013b). It is part of a larger trend of hospitals carefully tracking quality outcomes across numerous indicators, the results of which enhance insurance payments, if positive (or depress, if negative), from both government and private insurers.

One other approach to cost savings attempted in recent years is worth mentioning here. For certain kinds of medical goods and services, such as the purchase of motorized wheelchairs, Medicare now requires prior authorization. Beginning in 2012 in select areas of the country, program enrollees have had to provide documentation that they indeed need the medical devices or services in question before Medicare will guarantee payment to the provider. The Government Accountability Office (2018a) analyzed these payment practices and concluded that prior authorization saved the program an estimated $1.9 billion between 2012 and 2018. Prior authorization is routinely used in the private insurance industry but has only been applied in the Medicare space to a limited extent. The general idea is to reduce unnecessary utilization and to prevent inappropriate payments. Naturally, anytime an obstacle such as prior authorization is put in place, no matter how minor, it will discourage some users from obtaining needed services. However, even with the limited implementation of this process under Medicare, the savings have been significant, and studies have not tended to find systematic evidence of needed services going unmet (Government Accountability Office 2018a). Taking motorized wheelchairs as one example, without such prior authorization in place, makers of these devices could direct-market their goods to Medicare enrollees and sell many of them (which typically retail for more than $1,000 each), and the Medicare program would have to pay, whether or not the patient in question actually needs or would benefit from owning one. Even with this requirement in place, however, online advertisements are plentiful, and they encourage seniors to talk with their doctors, who then fill out the required paperwork to clear the authorization requirement. Attempting to control unnecessary utilization of medical devices more generally, the Centers for Medicare and Medicaid Services in June 2018 applied for prior authorization requirements of 31 new durable medical devices, prosthetics, orthotics, and supplies (Government Accountability Office 2019a, 2019b).

Medicare's high and rising costs have long made it a target for reform proposals from across the political spectrum. This contemporary debate plays out in three major directions, each explained below. First, some advocates claim that Americans should maintain Medicare's status quo, honoring the commitments that lawmakers have made to seniors and long-term disabled individuals under current law and ensuring that reliable funding streams remain in place to avoid shortages that would force more deficit spending than the federal government engages in already. A second line of argument goes that Congress should offer a Medicare-like public insurance option for those persons who cannot afford health insurance on the private market. Presumably, this would operate in competition with private insurance and would, therefore, experience significant political resistance from the for-profit insurance industry, though the idea also enjoys considerable public support. A third option, this one coming from the conservative end of the spectrum, calls for greater reliance on the private health insurance market. This approach calls for a shift away from Medicare's entitlement status to a voucher system that would provide Medicare-eligible persons with a credit applicable to purchases of private insurance. Beyond allowing individuals to purchase policies that best suit their particular needs, a key assumption behind this school of thought is that the flood of consumers searching for the best insurance policies would stimulate competition and drive down prices. This voucher—or premium-support model, as it is often called—has been the topic of considerable debate since the 1990s, with its latest round being pushed by U.S. House Speaker Paul Ryan during his time in office in the 2010s.

Beyond these broad approaches, many Democrats have called for expanding Medicare to all Americans. Vermont Senator and 2020 presidential candidate Bernie Sanders is the most prominent of these advocates, though others, including Massachusetts Senator Elizabeth Warren, also have endorsed this approach. Representative Pramila Jayapal of Washington State has introduced a Medicare for All bill in the U.S. House. The idea of Medicare for All is complex and will be explained separately as the next major controversy in this chapter.

Addressing Medicare's Budget, Option 1: Protect the Status Quo

Building on the strong public approval of current Medicare, opponents of liberal reforms to the program have made the case that Congress must keep the commitments it has made in law and that to expand eligibility to Americans other than the aged and disabled will necessarily undermine Congress's ability to keep those promises. Advocates who take this position, such as the Partnership for America's Health Care Future, typically argue that to extend coverage to younger people will boost program expenses without necessarily increasing the taxes paid into the Hospital Insurance Trust Fund. One version of this argument points out that guaranteeing new recipients' health insurance at individuals aged below 65, an idea sometimes referred to as a Medicare buy-in plan, will encourage these people to retire early or simply to work less, depriving Medicare of needed tax revenue. They argue that making more of the population eligible for Medicare will burden providers, especially hospitals who already have to deal with Medicaid patients. For others, taking the public position of *protecting Medicare* is part of a broader strategy to oppose further government involvement in health care provision.

To the significant degree that Medicare's HI Trust Fund is projected to run short on funds within a decade, a looming imbalance is ignored in protecting the status quo. Reducing expenditures alone is unlikely to solve the problem, since that would require deep cuts between now and 2025, the year that the HI Fund is projected to fail to meet its full obligations (Medicare Trustees 2019). A payroll tax rate hike could also address the problem, though this would almost certainly pose a political challenge for Republican members of Congress. A third option is to draw more money from the federal government's general revenue, though this would deprive other lines of programming and would likely just be added to the federal budget deficit, which is already estimated to exceed $1 trillion in FY 2020 (Congressional Budget Office 2019).

All of this is to say that programmatic changes could be very useful to both trim expenditures and raise revenue. Of course, merely doing nothing will not address this problem.

Addressing Medicare's Budget, Option 2: Adopt a Public Insurance Option

Many progressive advocates have called for the government to sell insurance to those who cannot afford the prices on the private market. For instance, the Democratically controlled U.S. House of Representatives included a public option in an early version of what later became the Affordable Care Act of 2010. Because the Senate was not willing to support this, this provision did not survive the reconciliation of the two chambers' versions. However, this idea has been a popular one over recent years in progressive circles. Former Vice-President and 2020 presidential candidate Joe Biden has supported this provision, for instance.

A financially self-sustaining public insurance option would be able to offer prices below those offered on the commercial market. The federal government, of course, operates as a non-profit organization, facing no multimillion salaries or bonuses to be paid to executive officers and no payments to be made to shareholders. Sidestepping profit concerns, beyond this, a public option would raise many issues that Congress would need to settle. Perhaps chief among them would be how to set prices and by how much these prices would undercut prevailing rates on the commercial market. For a public option to not underprice the commercial market would be to fail to live up to the chief purpose of such a system. Even if government rates were only slightly lower than prevailing commercial rates, this would have the effect of pressuring the for-profits to become more efficient in the pursuit of sustaining their market share. This much could benefit a wide variety of stakeholders.

The issue of market share is perhaps the most salient political question here. If Congress were to aggressively promote this insurance, it could effectively ruin the private health insurance industry. This prospect unsettles many Americans who value their current insurance arrangement, most of whom receive their insurance from their own or a family member's employer. A further set of questions has to do with how widely available a public insurance option would be. For instance, would access to government-sponsored insurance be means-tested? If so, how broadly available would this be? To borrow a reference point from the Affordable Care Act, perhaps families or individuals could be granted access to this option only if they were unable to purchase private insurance for less than a specific portion of their annual income. (The ACA used a threshold of 8%, though the penalty for not carrying health insurance was eliminated effective January 2019, so this threshold is no longer relevant.) If access to this option, or uptake by those who actually enrolled, skewed toward those with higher-than-average health care needs, taxpayers would be responsible to fund a program with a built-in adverse selection problem, meaning subscribers' premiums might not pay enough to cover their claims, depending on the premiums collected.

To borrow a second potential reference point from the ACA, purchases on a public option market could be limited to those who do not already have insurance through their employer and might even exclude persons who should be covered by their employers under an employer mandate. The ACA's employer mandate applies to firms with more than 50 workers and penalizes such employers who decline to offer health insurance. The penalty is triggered when one of those employees obtains insurance through the online Marketplace, a purchase that involves a federal tax subsidy. Leveraging the employer mandate concept would be a way not only to limit the scope of a public option but also to pressure employers to cover individuals who work for them.

In addition to questions about the impact of a public option for the insurance industry, this also raises concerns for medical providers. Because between one-third and one-half of the client load for the average hospital is currently on Medicare, financially healthy hospitals can absorb the loss associated with these low reimbursements. However, if the percentage of Medicare customers were to significantly increase, many hospitals would be unable to balance their budgets. The number of hospitals that closed in recent years provides a caution about a policy shift that would aggravate the financial strain under which they operate, particularly, though not exclusively, in rural areas. From 2010 to early 2019, fully 102 rural hospitals closed, nearly all due to financial problems, and nearly one-fifth of the remaining rural hospitals are facing serious financial risk, according to recent studies (Ellison 2019; Mosley and DeBehnke 2019). From a purely pragmatic perspective, whatever form a public option would assume, it would need to account for dwindling and aging populations in rural areas and the tremendous financial strain this places on care providers. Maintaining viable reimbursement rates would be essential, though again, this works against the urge to save money by putting downward pressure on premiums and payment levels to providers.

From a political perspective, proponents of a public insurance option frame this idea as a mechanism to offer people an affordable insurance option. On the other hand, opponents tend to critique this as an opening move toward a single-payer health insurance system, one that sooner or later would see the government undercutting the private market. Either way, proponents would surely encounter fierce resistance from the private insurance industry, as unlike the ACA's subsidies for purchases of health coverage, a public option would significantly depress private insurance sales.

Addressing Medicare's Budget, Option 3: Adopt a Premium-Support Model

Premium support is a broad term referring to a system under which government payments would subsidize private insurance purchases. In this particular context, premium support would give such credits to Medicare enrollees in lieu of the traditional coverage they have received since the inception of the program. This credit could work in a number of ways. It could be a fixed dollar amount per year. Alternatively, it could pay a percentage of the average private insurance plan costs for a given year, and this would likely be adjusted for different states or regions of the country to compensate for significant price differences. Most commentators also agree that benefits would need to be risk-adjusted to account for the widely differing health statuses of the enrollees (see Congressional Budget Office 2013 for a brief analysis).

The primary goal of a premium-support model would be to allow Congress to more readily control Medicare expenditures, in comparison to the open-ended entitlement of the current Medicare program. Beyond such a limited credit, beneficiaries would need to decide how much of their own money they want to spend for greater coverage. This arrangement would infuse some degree of price competition into the Medicare market, as insurance plans and medical provider groups would configure their plans to appeal to enrollees. Depending on how the insurance companies were to structure their cost-sharing provisions—co-payments, coinsurance, deductibles, and the like—this could encourage beneficiaries to become more cost-conscious as they utilize services, though the evidence on these likely impacts is mixed (Jost 2007). Premium support is similar to a defined contribution retirement plan, meaning the federal government would define how much it would spend on any single beneficiary rather than promising beneficiaries that it will cover all of their medical expenses. Fundamentally, this approach is based on the premise that seniors can do better for themselves by buying a plan that suits their particular needs rather than asking taxpayers to support a one-size-fits-all program.

The idea of premium support arose from the thinking that went into the proposed Clinton plan of the early 1990s. This was part of what was called a managed competition approach to health insurance financing that would have blended government-orchestrated competition among for-profit insurers (Enthoven 1980). Although these ideas were initially developed by policy thinkers who were associated with a Democratic administration, Congressional Republicans and others have proposed premium support for Medicare since the turn of the 21st century. House Speaker Paul Ryan advocated this shift during his time in office. Most recently, House Republicans proposed this as part of their fiscal year 2017 budget resolution, though this did not become law (Jacobson and Neuman 2016). At the time, the Congressional Budget Office estimated this proposal would save Medicare $537 billion over its first decade (National Committee to Preserve Social Security and Medicare 2018). A large part of the appeal of premium support for fiscal conservatives is that it would end one of the three largest entitlements currently in operation (Medicaid and Social Security being the other two) and would give Congress a more concrete spending target each year rather than promising to pay whatever charges Medicare beneficiaries and their providers rack up.

If Congress were to transition Medicare to a premium-support model, the federal payment toward individuals' insurance policies could be determined in various ways. For instance, the payment could be based on an average cost for insurance, such as average at the community level, state level, or regional level. Individuals' credits would need to be risk-adjusted, meaning that chronically ill persons would receive a larger credit, since their insurance premiums would be higher, assuming insurers were permitted to price plans according to specific individuals' needs, a process called individual experience rating. To not risk-adjust would place premiums out of reach for chronically ill people who are not also wealthy. However, even with such variation in the credits, insurers would likely seek to cherry-pick the healthiest subscribers if companies were not required to issue policies to all persons who wanted to purchase them. As one pair of experts on the subject put it, "Successful cherry-picking is privately profitable but socially wasteful, as costly enrollees will eventually be covered somewhere else in the system," such as at charity clinics of hospital emergency departments (Aaron and Lambrew 2008, 76). Given that a very small percentage of Medicare enrollees typically account for about one-half of all Medicare expenditures (5% of users accounted for 48% of spending in 2002), some sort of risk-adjustment would be necessary to entice insurers and Medicare beneficiaries to come to agreements on insurance purchases (Aaron and Lambrew 2008). Medicare Advantage already engages in risk-adjustment, based on age and past health service use, so this idea would not be novel to insurers.

As it turns out, there is quite a bit of debate about whether or not premium support would actually save the government money. Fundamentally, the question is whether insurers would collude to put upward pressure on prices, which would drive up federal payments (assuming these payments are tied to average premium costs or some similar benchmark), or whether insurers would instead engage in robust competition. A major determinant of this would be the number and type of insurance plans offered in each state or region. If the experience of the ACA is indicative, especially in rural states, the number of competing plans in any given area may lag.

Setting federal payments could involve either a fixed dollar amount that beneficiaries would receive each month or year in the form of a voucher (though many advocates avoid the term "voucher" due to its negative connotation) or at a percentage of insurance costs. Seniors would then be free to shop around for the insurance policy that best suits them. Alternatively, the value of the voucher could be tied to some economic index, such as the consumer price index, or to average wages, though because health care costs rise faster than either of these two particular indices, this would mean the voucher would lose purchasing power over time. When House Speaker Ryan proposed his premium-support plan, he wanted to connect the rise of payments over time to the inflation rate, which would have had the effect of eroding its purchasing power over time since the medical inflation rate is higher than the overall inflation rate. This strategy would escalate out-of-pocket costs for enrollees over time. Beyond this issue, providing credits, either as a percentage of premiums or as a fixed dollar amount, would mean that seniors with modest income would gravitate toward minimalist policies, and those with more income would tend to purchase more comprehensive coverage. This unevenness of coverage would be a fundamental departure from Medicare's long-standing formulation of providing the same benefits for all beneficiaries, regardless of income.

The matter of rising out-of-pocket costs poses a political problem for premium-support advocates. By design, those who desire health care spending to be more market-oriented explicitly want to see out-of-pocket expenses rise as part of making consumers more cost-conscious (Herzlinger 1997). However, this can be a difficult sales pitch to make as part of a campaign for elective office, and some politicians attempt to blur the implications of moving in a more market-oriented direction. For instance, in 2016, candidate Donald Trump promised voters that his ACA replacement plan would not only be "great" but also reduce out-of-pocket expenses. Forcing people to be cost-conscious while reducing their individual liability is (arguably, perhaps) impossible (Woolhandler and Himmelstein 2017). In any case, in 2013, the Congressional Budget Office analyzed projected costs for beneficiaries under a premium-support framework and concluded that for those who would remain in a plan that mimics traditional Medicare, out-of-pocket costs would rise regardless of whether federal payments were tied to the average plan cost or the cost of less expensive plans on the market (Congressional Budget Office 2013). If out-of-pocket costs were to rise significantly, this could lead to seniors pressuring Congress to add protections to cap this exposure, which in turn would at least partially undermine any savings generated by the adoption of premium support in the first place (Jacobson and Neuman 2016).

One other difficulty of moving to a premium-support model would be the transition from today's traditional Medicare to some new arrangement. Most advocates have proposed a phased transition, with Americans under some age, such as 55, being directed into a premium-support future and those over this age being grandfathered into either traditional Medicare or a Medicare Advantage plan. After all, people need time to plan financially for their future medical care (Neuman and Jacobson 2017). Setting the age threshold for who gets grandfathered and who does not would be a difficult political maneuver. There may emerge other considerations about who is allowed to continue on traditional Medicare and who is not. Congress might need to give special consideration to the chronically ill, for instance. This is a significant concern since the very ill account for a large share of overall Medicare spending. Specifically, in a typical year the top 10 percent of Medicare users account for a majority of all fee-for-service Medicare dollars spent (Potetz et al. 2011). For individuals in this category, giving them a voucher to purchase insurance may not get them very far if their premiums are risk-adjusted.

As with many policy proposals, the details of a shift to a premium-support framework for Medicare would involve many difficult political compromises. Beyond this, the fundamental question of whether Americans want to abandon the universal guarantee of coverage for all seniors would need to be settled, in addition to the highly contestable claim that such a move would save taxpayers a significant amount of money.

Problem #2: Building Medicare for All Would Pose Multiple Challenges

Over the past several years, Americans have heard a great deal of discussion of some form of a single-payer health care system. While *single payer* can mean different things, the core element would be government provision of health insurance for everyone, regardless of age, income, employment, or other personal situation. What the term single payer leaves unsettled is the matter of whether or not private insurance would also be available, among other points of contention.

Most developed nations use some form of a single-payer system, though they vary based on the degree of involvement of sub-national units of government, funding systems, the particulars of coverage, among other dimensions. To take a familiar model, Canada guarantees universal coverage for all, administers the plans at the provincial level, and allows citizens who want broader insurance coverage or faster access to purchase a supplemental private insurance policy. About 70 percent of Canadians do so, which allows them to access the many private providers. In contrast, the United Kingdom centralizes its single-payer system more, with the National Health Service owning or employing a greater portion of the providers than is the case in Canada. However, even in the United Kingdom, it is possible to purchase what is called voluntary insurance as a supplement to the broad public insurance made available to all who are ordinarily resident in the country (Johnson et al. 2018).

In the United States, when advocates call for Medicare for All, they may or may not be proposing an end to private insurance. Vermont Senator Bernie Sanders and Representative Jayapal want to give the federal government a monopoly over health insurance, effectively decimating the for-profit insurance industry (see Sanders' bill S. 1804 in the 115th Congress). Others would be content to extend Medicare (or a Medicare-like program) universally while allowing private insurance to remain available for those who desire to keep it. This latter approach may be appealing to workers in large firms, for instance, those who have negotiated high-coverage insurance plans with their employers and want to maintain their access to preferred providers. Those who want to eliminate private insurance typically argue that doing so will eliminate excessive national spending on health care attributable to profit-seeking and expensive overhead administrative costs. By one estimate, some two million Americans are employed processing private insurance claims. Many of those jobs would disappear under a Medicare for All or a public option arrangement (Johnson 2019).

Over Medicare's more than half century of experience, Congress has steadfastly refused to change the eligibility age from its original 65, though lawmakers have broadened the definition of disability, extending coverage, for instance, to persons with chronic kidney disease. To make Medicare, or something like it, available to many more Americans would, as referenced above, pose sweeping consequences for patients and their medical providers. Doing so would not only eliminate the insurance coverage gap experienced by 28 million Americans (as of 2019), but would also ensure that everyone could enjoy a basic minimum of coverage, which would help eliminate the dramatic cross-group differences in everything from dental hygiene to vaccinations and prenatal services, to premature mortality. These differences are particularly pronounced when comparing across racial groups (Smedley et al. 2003). Depending on its structure, services would become either free or very affordable at the point of service. At the system level, the cost-containment strategies put in place by the federal government would get a good deal of traction, as opposed to inconsistent efforts seen in our current system that is fragmented across states and numerous private insurers and provider networks. A single national system would certainly simplify billing procedures for medical providers. The adoption of the Sanders plan would also relieve state and local governments of a great deal of fiscal responsibility, although Medicaid would likely continue to cover the bulk of expensive and long-term nursing home care.

Of course, a move to Medicare for All would require a large increase in federal taxes. The Congressional Budget Office (Holahan et al. 2016) estimated that Senator Sanders' bill (S. 1804) would cost approximately $32 trillion over its first 10 years. Other analysts have developed similar estimates (Blahous 2018). The framing of this issue could proceed in a couple of ways. First, if one considers that this amount is less than Americans will spend on the combination of public and private health networks and that efficiencies can be achieved by streamlining the system's administration, this proposal sounds reasonable. Americans with health insurance might console themselves, considering that the taxes paid for such a system could amount to less than what they currently pay to their private insurers. On the other hand, many Americans will object to this number of dollars passing through their government's hands and might dwell on images of inefficiency and waste. Objections to paying higher taxes have been key obstacles for health policy proposals because of the way this maps on to objections about big government (Oberlander 2003). In fact, a July 2019 public opinion poll by the Kaiser Family Foundation reveals that when the idea of "too much government involvement in health care" is associated with a Medicare for All proposal, public support falls from a solid majority, approximately 65 percent, to something closer to 40 percent (Kaiser Family Foundation 2019b).

There would also be other challenges. Apart from the costs to taxpayers, a shift to a Medicare for All framework would severely limit hospitals' ability to adjust their payment balances against their patient mix, since they would become almost entirely dependent on a single payment schedule. Finally, the Department of Health and Human Services would need to expand its administrative capacity over a short period of time to implement this program. Critics have pointed this out—though one should consider that during Medicare's first year more than 19 million seniors were enrolled—with all this being accomplished prior to the age of computers.

The Sanders' proposal for Medicare for All leaves significant discretion to the secretary of the Department of Health and Human Services (Keith and Jost 2017). As written, the bill would allow assistance to be available to all residents of the United States, potentially even to undocumented immigrants. It would cover a range of services and would prohibit private insurers from covering the same services (Holahan et al. 2016). It would end the ACA's online marketplaces, the Federal Employees Health Benefits Program, and the TRICARE for Life program for military retirees. Most services would no longer be covered under the traditional Medicare program, Medicaid, or the Children's Health Insurance Program. In this last category, exceptions would include services for people who were inpatients or were receiving extended care during the transition from the current system to this new one or for people in need of services not covered by the new arrangement. The Sanders bill would ban cost sharing, with the exceptions of a new Medicaid long-term care program, and prescription drugs. An annual $200 limit on out-of-pocket for drugs would take effect, and balance billing would be banned. HHS would annually negotiate prices for drugs, devices, and assistive equipment.

The funding for the Sanders plan would come from an income-based payroll tax, presumably (but not explicitly) a progressive tax, with elevated rates for higher-income individuals.

Because this system would eliminate jobs in the insurance industry, the proposal also includes a funding stream to help these displaced workers learn skills to aid them in their transitions to other occupations. Just as Medicare does not cover long-term nursing home care now, neither would it under the Sanders plan. States would be required to use Medicaid to cover long-term care, nursing home care, home health services, and rehabilitative services. It would also require states to use Medicaid to cover inpatient psychiatric care for those under age 21. The act also calls for a public insurance option for use during the transitional phase.

Skeptics have questioned whether the Sanders plan would save money (Blahous 2018). Sanders' vision of Medicare for All is appealing to many because it is based on the assumption that the current schedule of payments to providers would remain largely unchanged. However, if all services for all patients were paid at these rates, most hospitals would face even greater financial strains than they currently do. Complicating this scenario, the Sanders bill envisions Medicare cuts for doctors at approximately 30 percent and those for hospitals at 40 percent (Holahan et al. 2016). Even if such cuts were not built into legislation that became law, providers would struggle with the current level of payments. The 87 cents paid on each dollar actually spent by hospitals on Medicare patients, compared unfavorably to the $1.45 paid on average by private insurance plans, casts in sharp relief the importance of a critical mass of private-pay patients, which help balance hospitals' budgets. If private insurance payments essentially disappear, their subsidizing effect would vanish along with them, leading most hospitals to operate at a loss (American Hospital Association 2018). Obviously, this is not sustainable.

Public opinion polls conducted during 2019 and the spring of 2020 found qualified support for Medicare for All. As with most issues, the framing of the question matters a great deal. When asked if they approve or disapprove of allowing Americans to buy into Medicare if they choose, about two-thirds of respondents expressed support for such a plan. During this time, solid majorities, approximately 60 percent, also told pollsters that adopting Medicare buy-in was a high priority. However, when reminded that this would lead to tax increases or that Medicare for All would eliminate private insurance plans, Americans were nearly evenly divided between supporting and opposing this. This qualified public support—not only liking the idea of government insurance but also finding a minority portion of those supporters who express reluctance to cede their private plans—prominently played out between Senator Bernie Sanders and former Vice-President Joe Biden during the Democratic primaries in early 2020. Regardless of how this issue cleaves the electorate in the 2020 cycle, this is very likely to persist as a concern among Democrats in the near future.

Problem #3: Medicare Advantage Is Not Generating the Expected Savings

Medicare Advantage is the managed care version of Medicare. Created under Part C as a component of the Balanced Budget Act of 1997 and initially called Medicare+Choice, this system pays private insurers to cover the medical needs of individuals who enroll in this alternative to traditional Medicare. Approximately, one-third of all Medicare beneficiaries were covered by a Medicare Advantage plan as of 2018. This has been the most significant development in the history of private contracting for payments in the history of Medicare. The creation of this component of Medicare was expected to generate savings through more efficient matching of groups of plan subscribers to groups of contracted medical providers. This same logic drove the rapid expansion of managed care systems since the 1990s in the private insurance market. The problem, however, is that on the Medicare side of things this adoption of managed care plans has not generated the expected savings in large part because of the limited competition at play among private insurers who participate in Medicare Advantage plans.

Medicare Advantage plans have ballooned in popularity among seniors over the past decade, mainly because they allow enrollees to cap their annual out-of-pocket expenses, something traditional Medicare does not do. Further, these plans generally cover a broader range of services than does the traditional program, often including optical and prescription drugs at little or no extra expense. In exchange for these benefits, Medicare Advantage enrollees commit to a limited network of providers, much like anyone else who is covered by a health maintenance organization.

When policy makers first created this program, private insurers were to be paid a capitated rate that was 95 percent of the average annual cost for Medicare recipients in a given county. Insurers would assume full risk, meaning they would be responsible to cover whatever health services would normally be covered by Medicare's Parts A and B among their subscribers. This 5 percent reduction in payment was based on the assumption that a managed care framework could deliver goods and services more efficiently than the traditional fee-for-service Medicare model. Policy makers expected that managed care would generate significant savings and that these savings would be shared by the insurers, providing them an incentive to participate in this portion of the Medicare program (Zarabozo 2000).

As part of the Balanced Budget Act, Congress adjusted the basis for payments, setting a floor based on rural areas, where it could be difficult to attract insurers. Further attempting to entice insurers into thinly covered areas, the Medicare Modernization Act of 2003 increased payments nationwide. Building on this in one more step, in 2006 payments came to be based on individually adjusted factors, such as age and health status. This individual experience rating helps insurers closely assess their risks and bid their coverage accordingly.

Layered atop this, each county in the United States is assigned a benchmark reimbursement level by Medicare. Insurers bid to offer coverage in each county where they want to participate, and if their bid is less than the benchmark amount, the difference is shared between Medicare and the insurer, with most of this savings—referred to as a rebate—going to the insurer and the remainder going back to Medicare. If the bid is higher than the county-level benchmark, the extra cost is passed on to subscribers, who in these cases are typically individuals who are seeking a higher level of coverage than is typical and who are willing to pay for it. In the cases of plans below the benchmarks, insurers are permitted to apply part of this rebate to cover administrative expenses (which in turn helps boost profitability), while the rest must be applied to improving service coverage. This latter category typically involves broadening the scope of services covered, such as optical services and prescription drugs, and reducing cost-sharing obligations, such as co-payments. In recent years only about one-half of the portion rebated to insurers was passed on to enrollees, while insurers recouped the remainder (Neuman and Jacobson 2018). The Centers for Medicare and Medicaid Services studied this pattern in the mid-2000s and found that on average 25 percent of the difference between the county-level benchmark and the bid was returned to Medicare and 75 percent was rebated to insurers (Duggan et al. 2016). The size of these rebates has grown in recent years. Between 2015 and 2018, they more than doubled, from a total of $3 billion to $6.3 billion. This growth represents not only an increase in the per person amount but also the large increase in the number of enrollees in Medicare Advantage (Jacobson et al. 2018). In an effort to maximize profits, the insurance industry would like these benchmarks to be based on higher-intensity users than has been the case in recent years (America's Health Insurance Plans 2019). This calculation method will likely be contested as the ranks of Medicare Advantage subscribers continue to grow.

The numbers of seniors enrolled in Medicare Advantage is indeed poised to continue significantly steep growth. Insurers experience it as profitable, the Trump Administration has pushed the program aggressively, and moving enrollees on to quasi-private insurance positions this population for a potential shift to a voucher system. An October 2019 executive order from the Trump White House eased the way to enrolling more seniors in Medicare Advantage by allowing automatic enrollment of individuals into private plans, among other changes (Center for Medicare Advocacy 2019). Once a critical mass of older Americans come to think of their government insurance as private, which it is not, it would be a politically easier lift to entice them into a funding arrangement where the government's financial obligation is closed-ended, as a voucher system would have it. Progressive groups have articulated this complaint for years.

From private insurers' perspective, they see in Medicare Advantage the opportunity to offer very efficient coverage plans, allowing them to recoup significant rebates, a large portion of which effectively become profit. This should also generate savings for taxpayers, as a portion of the savings accrue to the Medicare program. However, such efficiencies are more difficult to generate than policy makers initially thought, especially while also striving to maintain high levels of quality care. At their worst in 2009, the average Medicare Advantage plan cost 114 percent of what it cost the average person on traditional Medicare. Some greater efficiencies have been realized in the intervening years. These have been catalyzed in part by greater competition between insurance plans, and reductions have been made to Medicare reimbursement schedules pursuant to the Affordable Care Act. By 2018, the average Medicare Advantage enrollee cost the Medicare program 101 percent of the cost of average person on traditional Medicare. Hence, program savings still prove difficult to achieve. Reimbursement reductions alone, such as those already made and still to be put into effect under the ACA, to the tune of an estimated $156 billion between 2013 and 2022, will not likely fundamentally alter the challenge of simultaneously saving money, broadening service coverage, and maintaining quality (Neuman and Jacobson 2018; Duggan et al. 2016).

One way to think about the core of this difficulty is that Congress has created a program that is increasingly popular with Medicare beneficiaries, evidenced by a tripling of enrollment over the past decade, but that does not powerfully enough incentivize for-profit insurers to steer patients and providers toward highly efficient and high quality care. When benchmark payment levels have risen, this has drawn more insurers into specific markets. While this enrolls more seniors in coverage plans they like, higher benchmarks limit potential program savings. Further, in these circumstances insurers have been found to spend significantly more money on expenses such as marketing instead of improved patient care. The evidence is mixed as to whether increased payments consistently lead to improved quality. Thus, it seems that when Medicare pays more, this mainly benefits insurers rather than patients or providers (Duggan et al. 2016).

Part of the problem is that many Medicare recipients are unable or unwilling to adequately compare health plans to optimize their coverage. Enrollments have been described as "sticky," with seniors not acting like savvy shoppers who would pick the most appropriate coverage, given their individual circumstances (Neuman and Jacobson 2018). If they could do so, they would likely gravitate toward less expensive plans, which in turn would save money for the Medicare program. Analogous to the often complicated long-distance calling plans in the 1980s and 1990s, the wide variation in Medicare Advantage plans makes it difficult for seniors to do comparison shopping. One reform idea would be for Congress to impose a simplifying framework on these plans. However, this would likely run into resistance from the many employers and labor unions that sponsor group plans for their retirees. Such plans allow the sponsor to pay a portion of the premium while limiting any further exposure to risk on behalf of their former employees. Seniors, despite the evidence that they do not shop around as carefully as they should, might also resist a push toward standardizing. Most of them have many plans to choose from: 21 on average as of 2018, more in urban areas. Some evidence suggests that this competition may be exerting downward pressure on prices (Neuman and Jacobson 2018). Those persons living in rural counties generally have many fewer choices. Nationwide, three insurers account for most Medicare Advantage enrollees. As of 2018, United Healthcare covers 25 percent, Humana another 17 percent, and BCBS picks up an additional 13 percent (Jacobson et al. 2018).

One other possible point of reform has to do with the annual out-of-pocket limits imposed on Medicare Advantage plans. Since 2011, these have been limited by law. Depending on whether one enrolls in a preferred provider organization or a more typical health maintenance organization, these limits can vary. However, they do not exceed $6,700 per year for in-network providers (Jacobson et al. 2018). This level of out-of-pocket spending has held more or less steady since 2011. Congress could adjust these amounts, which would reduce one important dimension that distinguishes Medicare Advantage from traditional Medicare, recalling that the latter has no out-of-pocket limits on enrollees' obligations.

The near-term future of Medicare Advantage seems to be not only one of growing popularity but also of tremendous expense. It is estimated that these plans will account for 42 percent of the Medicare population by 2028, compared to approximately one-third currently. Its costs are expected to rise from $200 billion in 2017 to $580 billion by 2028. This does not count prescription drug costs (Neuman and Jacobson 2018). If, as some observers note, Medicare Advantage continues to over-pay many of its participating insurers, this will cost Medicare a couple of hundred billion dollars over the coming decade (Kronick 2017). It is ironic that a program that Congress created to save money has ended up costing taxpayers significantly more.

Problem #4: Medicare Part D Is Not Getting Taxpayers the Best Value for Their Money

When President George W. Bush signed into law the Medicare Prescription Drug, Improvement, and Modernization Act in

December 2003, he welcomed a variety of changes to Medicare, though the one that attracted the greatest attention was the addition of a prescription drug program, or Part D, which took effect in 2006. This added benefit allows Medicare beneficiaries to purchase a modestly priced drug plan that is suited to their particular needs and to enjoy considerable insurance coverage in exchange. Individual premiums averaged about $35 per month in 2019. Enrollment in Part D is not mandatory for Medicare beneficiaries, though to not enroll, in absence of other prescription drug coverage, typically involves a financial penalty when one finally gets around to enrolling. Initially, the coverage came in tiers that were dramatically different enough that beneficiaries experienced a coverage gap, referred to as the doughnut hole, when their annual drug expenses amounted to between $3,600 and $5,100 (see Chapter 1 for discussion). This gap was gradually closed in 2020 under the Affordable Care Act, though until that occurred a significant portion of enrollees faced thousands of dollars of drug expenses each year despite being enrolled in Part D coverage.

Unlike the political discourse surrounding the enactment of Medicare Part C and the expectation of cost savings, the enactment of Part D was generally framed as a coverage expansion that would cost taxpayers hundreds of millions of dollars over its first decade (Oliver et al. 2004). Some provisions were built into the law that would encourage savings by driving down drug prices. However, these mechanisms have not consistently worked to keep per-person drug spending below the nation's overall inflation rate. First, a rule was created that requires drug makers to issue rebates to Medicare that help defray government expenditures. Medicaid has used such a rebate provision for years, and this has saved the federal and state governments considerable amounts of money under this program. The rebates under Medicare, however, are more modest, so they have driven down the government's net costs less than on the Medicaid side (Congressional Budget Office 2014). Beyond this, private insurers who participate in the Part D program can leverage lower drug prices through competition in the bids they secure from drug makers, and this has been useful in containing costs below what they would have been, in the absence of this provision. However, it would be a serious misrepresentation to portray Part D as primarily a money-saving move for the federal government. This is an expensive program. For instance, in 2013 the federal government spent $50 billion on Part D, net of premiums paid and payments received from states associated with individuals who are eligible for both Medicare and Medicaid (Congressional Budget Office 2014). Hence, the question of whether HHS is doing as well for itself it could is part of a lively debate. This issue has received heightened attention in recent years as drug prices have risen dramatically.

At the heart of this debate is Part D's noninterference clause, a single sentence found in the Medicare Modernization Act. This clause states that the Secretary of the Department of Health and Human Services "may not interfere with the negotiations between drug manufacturers and pharmacies and PDP sponsors, and may not require a particular formulary or institute a price structure for the reimbursement of covered Part D drugs." This means that HHS cannot use its bulk purchasing power to negotiate or set prices for Part D. Regardless of the fact that government expenditures for these benefits during its first decade were significantly less than initially projected, on the face of it, the noninterference clause has been part of a very lucrative deal for the pharmaceutical industry (Shih et al. 2016; Potter and Penniman 2016).

In search of a few more votes to win passage of the Medicare Modernization Act, House Speaker Dennis Hastert and other GOP leaders added this provision late in the legislative process in 2003 (Aaron and Lambrew 2008). To disallow HHS from negotiating or setting drug prices, it was framed, for the benefit of a few conservative Republican members who were reluctant to support the measure, as an assurance that the government officials would not be able to interfere with market dynamics. The irony, however, is that the new drug program also made

HHS the largest consumer in the market, and it put HHS in the position of essentially paying whatever the drug makers asked. In this sense, the noninterference clause is profoundly anticompetitive. Rebates paid by drug makers can essentially be canceled out whenever drug makers simply increase their bid price, something they do each summer when they submit their bids to HHS.

In contrast to this prohibition that limits HHS, four other federal government agencies that purchase large quantities of pharmaceuticals are permitted to negotiate prices. The Department of Defense, the Department of Veterans Affairs, the U.S. Public Health Service, and the Coast Guard are all allowed to leverage lower prices through their bulk purchasing power (Shih et al. 2016). This results in them enjoying preferential pricing and significant discounts (Government Accountability Office 2013a). Medicare is still a larger payer than any of these other agencies—The Big Four, as they are known in the pharmaceutical lobbying community—so freeing it to negotiate prices poses a significant threat to the lucrative deal that the drug industry enjoys under Part D.

For their part, the pharmaceutical industry argues that, on principle, the government should not be allowed to set prices and that the market should instead determine these. Further, the Pharmaceutical Research and Manufacturers of America (or PhRMA, as it is usually referred to), the industry's major lobbying group, insists that allowing HHS to negotiate prices would result in the money reverting to "the government" and not to Medicare recipients. PhRMA's press release of July 25, 2019, of course, does not discuss this in terms of the savings to taxpayers that would result from such a change (Pharmaceutical Research and Manufacturers of America 2019).

The issue of whether or not Part D operates efficiently tended to receive less attention in the early years of the program than it has in the 2010s. One issue has to do with how seniors tend to select plans. Because they face numerous options that cover a complex mix of drugs, research has found that many seniors seem to select myopically based on premium price rather than on the plan that best fits their needs (Abaluck and Gruber 2011). This results in many beneficiaries purchasing the wrong benefit plan. On the other hand, the program overall has cost taxpayers less than initially expected. According to a report by the Congressional Budget Office, in 2013 the program actually spent only 50 percent of what was expected. Competition among the plans offered was largely credited to the savings.

Beyond this competition, during its first few years of operation at least three other factors contributed to slowing inflation in per-person drug spending. First, many name brand drugs saw their patents expire, exposing them to generic competition, which fostered lower prices. Second, fewer new drugs came on the market during this time. The net effect is that the mix of drugs on the market shifted toward more generics, exerting downward pressure on prices overall. Third, enrollment in Part D was smaller than initially projected, amounting to only 12 percent of Medicare enrollees in 2012. This is in part due to the presence of employer- or union-based drug plans and the fact that beneficiaries must actively sign up for Part D if they want it, as opposed to enrollment being automatic (Government Accountability Office 2014).

If the noninterference clause were repealed, several questions would need to be addressed. HHS would need to adopt a transparent and consistently applied process for negotiating prices. Would it treat different drug makers differently, perhaps focusing more intense pressure on the makers of very expensive drugs, such as Sovaldi, the hepatitis C drug that has been marketed for $1,000 per pill or $84,000 for a course of treatment (LaMattina 2016)? On the other hand, would it focus greater pressure on the makers of drugs that are widely used and which have seen spikes in prices in the past few years, such as insulin or epinephrine? Would makers of drugs that have no competition be essentially immune from negotiating prices, since they can make a take-it-or-leave-it offer to the government?

Despite its problems, Medicare Part D has become an important program for those seniors who lack some other prescription drug plan, and such benefits, once granted, are notoriously difficult to curtail or eliminate. While the vast majority of Americans believe Medicare officials should be able to negotiate lower drug prices—86 percent in a February 2019 poll by the Kaiser Family Foundation—the intense pressure by the pharmaceutical industry will likely make this a challenge to reverse.

Problem #5: Low Medicaid Reimbursement Levels Limit Patient Choice and Medical Provider Participation

The effort to extend insurance coverage to millions of low-income families and individuals has historically been accomplished by lowering the reimbursement rates to medical providers, stretching the state and federal dollars to cover as many people as possible. The problem, of course, is that these low, and often very slow, payments to doctors, hospitals, and clinics typically limit these providers' willingness to see Medicaid patients. It is common that clinicians restrict the proportion of their patient mix who will use Medicaid as payment, as they need to preserve a larger percentage for those who bring larger payments, which effectively make up for the Medicaid-related payment deficit. The need for providers to maintain a patient mix that keeps the proportion of Medicaid patients low has a direct impact on the kinds of providers who are willing to take on new Medicaid patients, and this is particularly consequential at a time when the Affordable Care Act has broadened the number of Americans who seek to use Medicaid as their means of payment. Some 13 million additional people joined Medicaid between 2013 and 2018 (Holgash and Heberlein 2019). This expansion, unless accompanied by a rise in the number of clinicians willing to accept this as payment, will have an adverse effect on other Medicaid beneficiaries since spots for new patients will become scarcer.

Since the turn of the millennium, the percentage of physicians who accept Medicaid has declined slightly. In the late 1990s, only 13 percent of doctors reported no Medicaid revenue. This figure rose to 15 percent by 2004. More recent studies have found that while close to 70 percent of doctors' offices have some Medicaid patients, only about one-half of them have reported being willing to accept new Medicaid patients (Cunningham and May 2006; Holgash and Heberlein 2019). While the overall percentage shows only a slight change, a larger shift has occurred in the types of medical offices that accept Medicaid. Specifically, small clinics with either one or only a few physicians have curtailed their Medicaid patient load, as they have fewer private-pay patients to help subsidize the losses associated with public insurance. This has led to a growing concentration of Medicaid patients at the facilities that are willing to accept them. Those providers who are willing to see a large number of Medicaid patients tend to concentrate more in smaller metropolitan areas and rural settings (Cunningham and May 2006; Paradise 2017). Overall, when comparing across states and using data from 2016, Holgash and Heberlein (2019) found that Medicaid paid on average only 72 percent of what Medicare provided.

Attempts to understand which medical providers are most willing to accept Medicaid payment have led researchers to examine reimbursement levels, the speed at which those payments arrive, among other variables. Levels of reimbursement and the timeliness of payments vary considerably across states. For instance, working with data from 2006, Cunningham and O'Malley (2008) found that average reimbursement times ranged from a low of 37 days in Kansas to 115 days in Pennsylvania. Reimbursement levels also vary greatly across states. However, the search for simple explanations for acceptance rates has met with only limited success. Several studies have pointed out a noticeable but not particularly strong positive relationship between payment levels and the percentage of doctors who accept Medicaid. Holgash and Heberlein (2019) found a greater percentage of doctors being willing to take on new Medicaid patients when payment levels are set higher, though the relationship was neither strong nor consistent. Their analysis found that, on average, Medicaid acceptance rates rise by 0.78 percent for every one percentage point rise in payment rates. Beyond the matter of low payments, the bureaucratic hurdles encountered with Medicaid agencies frequently elicit complaints from doctors' office workers who dislike the complexity of administrative procedures involved in requesting payments, which consume valuable staff time.

As mentioned above, many hospital systems have worked diligently to try to streamline their operations enough to break even on Medicare-paid services. For most, this goal has been elusive, though with an aging population this is also becoming increasingly crucial. As difficult as this is for Medicare, this is virtually impossible with Medicaid patients and the small payments that providers receive for treating them.

Most of the political conversation about Medicaid payment rates has focused on their inadequacy. However, it is important to note that there are actually several different payment rates, depending on the system a state uses to cover a given sub-population. For instance, many states have shifted to managed care arrangements for some or all of their Medicaid populations, and these reforms have shown significant efficiencies. These payment systems have allowed states to cover growing portions of their residents over time while preventing the program from consuming significantly greater portions of their state budgets. Of course, a shift to managed care and its contracts with specific provider groups entails a loss of patient choice. This tendency is aggravated by the fact that many doctors' offices accept only a limited number of Medicaid patients to begin with. Other efforts have been made to tailor payments based on the specifics of various sub-populations. Various payment schedules range from the traditional fee-for-service rate that reimburses providers for each individual service to the managed care organization rate, which bundles services, to the

Indian Health Service rate, which bills per encounter with a clinician, not for each specific service (Centers for Medicare and Medicaid Services 2019).

The long-standing recognition that Medicaid reimbursements do not typically cover the cost of service delivery has been addressed in a provision of federal law that allows special payments to states, which are then passed on to hospitals that treat a higher than average number of Medicare patients. (Another part of this program involves payments associated with Medicare populations.) The Disproportionate Share Hospital Program (DSH), created in 1981, helps these hospitals balance their revenues in light of the substantial amount of uncompensated care associated with the Medicaid population. Due to a loophole in the initial version of the law, states used an accounting maneuver—sometimes referred to as bootstrapping—to wring many billions of dollars out of the U.S. Treasury during the late 1980s under this program. Because in the beginning the DSH program allowed states to draw down more than one federal dollar for each state dollar they added to their Medicaid budgets, many states leveraged payments from hospitals in order to make it appear that state governments had boosted their spending on the program, in turn drawing down more federal dollars, some of which were returned to the hospitals that had contributed funds in the first place. This accounting shuffle led to a dramatic rise in DSH payments, from $1.3 billion in 1990 to $17.7 billion in 1992. Congress responded, imposing limits on states, so as to ensure that the federal funds had to be justified by actual levels of uncompensated care. Despite these controls, which now must involve an independent yearly audit of the expenses, the DSH program still costs federal tax payers a great deal. During fiscal year 2017, a total of $18.1 billion in DSH payments were made, $7.7 in state funds, and $10.4 billion from the federal government (Medicaid and CHIP Payment Access Commission 2019). Various federal statutes passed since the creation of the ACA have slowed planned reductions to the

DSH payments. The statutory cuts will be $4 billion in 2020, rising to $8 billion annually from 2022 through 2025. The logic here is that fewer DSH payments will be needed since with the drop in the uninsured population hospitals will face fewer uncompensated costs.

Going forward, low Medicaid reimbursement levels will very likely remain below the actual cost of service delivery. Fixing this problem would involve upward adjustments at the state level, and since states have very limited legal ability to deficit spend, and almost no incentive to offer payments that are any higher than absolutely necessary to retain a critical mass of providers in the Medicaid market, the future of these payment systems seems quite unlikely to fundamentally change.

Problem #6: Medicaid Is Not a Sustainable Way to Cover Long-Term Nursing Home Care

When Congress created Medicare, most Democratic lawmakers assumed that this would be an initial step toward a universal care program; thus, it made sense to place long-term care coverage under Medicaid, based on the idea of sweeping it into a broader program later (Marmor 2003). That this evolution has not occurred leaves various services scattered about in ways that are complex and not user-friendly for beneficiaries, service providers, or governments. Medicare will pay for up to 100 days of skilled nursing home care per year, so this means that families whose members need long-term care must either tap into their own resources to pay for these services or turn to Medicaid, which will cover these services long term. As of 2019, a private-pay spot in a nursing facility usually cost at least $275 per day, or over $8,000 per month. In 13 of the states in 2019, the average monthly charge exceeded $10,000 (Ramsey 2019).

For middle-class people, making oneself eligible for Medicaid is a traumatic process. While state-by-state requirements vary, this generally involves spending down nearly all of one's liquid resources—savings and checking accounts, life insurance policies, retirement accounts, etc.—and dedicating those funds to one's medical care and ordinary living expenses. Merely giving away one's resources, for instance, to one's family, is not a permitted way to handle this transition. Forty-nine of the fifty states conduct a five-year lookback over one's finances to ensure that resources were spent on customary living expenses, health care, or advance funeral arrangements (California looks back over 30 months). Once on Medicaid, permitted cash reserves typically cannot exceed $2,000, and nearly all of one's monthly income must be paid to the nursing home, except $50–$100 per month to cover personal expenses.

While rendering oneself poor is traumatic for those seeking Medicaid assistance, neither does this payment method pose a particularly good outcome for nursing homes. The evidence suggests that most states set payment levels about as low as they can get away with, meaning they pay as little as a critical mass of nursing facilities would accept without refusing to accept Medicaid patients outright, though many do adopt this posture. This means that the number of beds available for Medicaid enrollees is limited in most communities. Better quality nursing homes generally limit their number of Medicaid beds to a small percentage; less elegant facilities will accept more.

While the variation in availability of Medicaid spots in nursing homes across communities is wide, this has become the single most common way for elderly Americans to cover these living arrangements. As of 2015, Medicaid was the primary payer for nearly two-thirds of nursing home residents nationwide, paying for 40 percent of all nursing home costs (Quadagno 2015). The pressures of low reimbursement rates and an aging population will test this tenuous balance in the years to come.

A survey of nursing homes in late 2017 found that Medicaid paid, on average, $206 per day, compared to $257 for private payers (Liberman 2018). Payments tend to be higher in urban than in rural areas. In many places, these payments are not enough to cover the cost of care, leading nursing home administrators to look to other payment modes, such as private pay and Medicare clients, to bridge the gap. One attempted solution has been to pass legislation at the state level to create dedicated funds to ensure adequate payment levels. This was attempted in Missouri in 2018. Lutheran Senior Services, an organization that operates several nursing homes, found that on average it costs $178 per day to care for a nursing home resident, yet Missouri only paid $153 under its Medicaid program, which is also called MO HealthNet (Parkins 2018). Missouri hiked its per diem payment by just $8 in 2018, though this did not close the gap between what Medicaid pays and what nursing homes spend on each patient (Centers for Medicare and Medicaid Services 2018).

A wave of nursing home closures, particular concentrated in rural areas, has caught the attention of facility administrators, families, legislators, and others in recent years. A 2019 *New York Times* story reported the closure or merger of 440 rural homes in the past decade (Healy 2019). While several factors are likely at play—including quality care violations, population loss in rural America, and shifts in the patient mix in many nursing homes—low Medicaid payments will continue to plague the long-term care industry and the families they serve.

Problem #7: The Medicaid Expansion under the ACA Has Been Uneven

When Congress passed the Affordable Care Act in 2010, a key provision was to expand the Medicaid program to cover millions of low- and modest-income Americans who cannot afford to purchase health insurance. Lawmakers found this route relatively easy, since it would build on an existing program with a long track record. The ACA's language called for all states to raise the income eligibility threshold from the federal poverty level (FPL) up to 133 percent of this level. Because Medicaid law allows 5 percent of a family's income to be ignored during eligibility determination, this effectively raised the new threshold to 138 percent of the FPL. Americans having income above this new threshold, up to 400 percent of the FPL, are able to receive a federal subsidy to purchase private insurance on exchanges created either by their home states or by the federal government. The passage of the last several years has provided clear evidence that access to health care services for low-income Americans has been significantly improved in those states that elected to expand their Medicaid programs (Government Accountability Office 2018c).

Lawmakers aimed to make this expansion inviting for states by including federal payment of 100 percent of the costs for the Medicaid expansion population starting in 2014 and extending through 2016, a figure set to taper to 90 percent in 2020. As it turned out, however, most Republican-controlled states objected, and when they and others sued the Obama Administration, they ultimately prevailed, winning in the Supreme Court in 2012. In the case of *National Federation of Independent Businesses v. Kathleen Sebelius*, the Court ruled that the mandated Medicaid expansion abused the fine balance of American federalism and that Congress lacked the authority to require states to expand this program that, since its inception, has been voluntary for states to operate. About one-half of the states proceeded with the expansion, while the others did not. What Democratic members of Congress initially envisioned to be a natural expansion of a long-standing program turned into an episode of protracted partisan warfare. Republican leaders in numerous states decided that it would be preferable to leave hundreds of millions of federal dollars on the table per state than to cooperate with Obamacare (Béland et al. 2016; Shaw 2017). The result has been that millions of Americans have gone without health insurance who could have been covered nearly entirely at federal expense. Specifically, those people with incomes above the thresholds for traditional Medicaid, yet below the 138 percent level at which people become eligible to shop for insurance on the online exchanges, fall into a coverage gap estimated to include some 2.5 million adults as of 2019, most of whom reside in a small number of southern states, mainly Texas, Florida, Georgia, and North Carolina (Kaiser Family Foundation 2019a). Children in families with income at these levels tend to be covered by the Children's Health Insurance Program.

The number of Americans finding themselves in this coverage gap would be much larger if not for the gradual movement of most Republican states to adopt some version of the Medicaid expansion between 2015 and 2018. While the politics of state by state adoptions are complex and varied, a central theme was the decision of conservative states to expand their Medicaid programs under federal waivers that permit them to add a veneer of private insurance-like features that allow state politicians to talk about Medicaid involving an element of personal responsibility. These provisions have included token premiums and co-payments, account statements showing personalized transaction records, and incentives for regular doctor visits and childhood vaccinations. The idea of hearing advocates tell the story is to ensure that enrollees have some "skin in the game" or that they experience some measure, however small, of personal accountability (Shaw 2017). In addition to these maneuvers, many Republican-controlled states have applied for federal waivers to allow them to attach work requirements and other eligibility restrictions to the program. The offer of such waivers by the Trump Administration piqued the interest of at least six more states to expand Medicaid during 2019 alone (Hayes et al. 2019).

These recent approvals now mean that the large majority of adults who could be eligible for the Medicaid expansion have found a way in to the program. This helps not only the recipients but also state budgets, since it takes the pressure off other public health programs as these individuals shift to Medicaid, and for this expansion population, the 10 percent of program costs that states will bear make up only a tiny portion of the average state's budget. While this much is considered good news by most involved, the 2.5 million who remain uncovered experience not only the lack of coverage themselves, which translates to significant trouble in finding willing care providers, but it also continues to aggravate the pattern of uncompensated care borne by health care providers, particularly hospital emergency departments in low-income areas. While it is impossible to predict if all states will eventually adopt the Medicaid expansion, the evidence from 2019 points toward this outcome. Federal waivers allowing states to give their welfare and Medicaid programs the imprimatur of homegrown and ideologically suitable appearances goes a long way toward making them palatable to erstwhile opponents. Arizona delayed until 1981 before it adopted Medicaid at all. The likely adoptions of the Medicaid expansion seem on track of progressing a bit faster than that.

Problem #8: Medicare Experiences a High Level of Improper Payments

The great complexity of the Medicare program leaves it vulnerable to high levels of improper payments to medical providers. These problems range from administrative errors, which can occur when medical providers inadvertently bill for services not rendered, to the overstatement of service intensiveness, to outright intentional fraud on the part of providers. According to the Government Accountability Office (2019a), CMS made improper payments in fiscal year 2017 estimated at $51.9 billion (out of about $706 billion in total program costs). Congress, through compelled testimony and a series of critical reports generated by the GAO, its watchdog agency, has pushed CMS over the past few years to seek improvements in some numerous areas of Medicare operations (Government Accountability Office 2018b). A spring 2019 GAO analysis found that CMS had made progress in some but not all of these areas. Although bundled payments encouraged by the Affordable Care Act have shifted the incentives in inpatient settings to focus on quality and efficiency rather than on the number of intensiveness of services, there is still a long way to go to aligning payments to providers with the actual goods and services rendered.

The problem of inappropriate payments persists under both traditional Medicare and Medicare Advantage plans. In 2016, the Government Accountability Office found that medical providers often file claims that are not substantiated by proper diagnoses (Government Accountability Office 2016). Specifically, the GAO found in its investigation that CMS improperly paid $14.1 billion to Medicare Advantage organizations in 2013. While the Centers for Medicare and Medicaid Services routinely conducts audits of Medicare Advantage contracts with insurers, through the 20-teens, it has established a record of not consistently looking where the bulk of the problems occurs. On examining CMS's 2011 audit of contracts and payments, the GAO concluded that CMS showed a poorly developed methodology for focusing on the contracts with the highest probability of improper payments. In particular, the GAO critiqued the audit, noting that only four of the 30 contracts reviewed showed particularly high risk for improper payments. Finally, the GAO concluded that the CMS lacked a concrete plan to remedy the problem. While one might argue that CMS should look at a variety of contracts, perhaps even a representative sample of them, the GAO's criticism for not focusing on the areas where problems are likely to be most prevalent is compelling. Stepping back to view improper Medicare payments more generally, it has long been recognized that these are common and that they amount to billions of dollars each year. In this respect, Medicare Advantage plans are not unique. Nonetheless, a concerted effort to improve accuracy, and to combat intentional fraud, is certainly warranted.

Looking at the problem of fraud specifically, this can be difficult for the CMS staff to detect; thus the agency has attempted to enlist the help of beneficiaries. Enrollees receive statements of payments made to providers on their behalf, and CMS encourages them to review these statements and report suspicious payments. The website of the Office of the Inspector General at HHS (the parent agency of the CMS) offers tips to help seniors detect fraud. In contrast, relying on its own resources, the department employs data analytics to spot suspicious billing patterns from providers, such as the Houston, Texas, physician convicted in federal court in October 2019 for fraudulently signing home health care plans, resulting in fraudulent payments between 2012 and 2016 amounting to $16 million. The home health services were either not needed, or not delivered, or both (Department of Justice 2019). Hundreds of other instances of fraud have been pursued by the Department of Health and Human Services in recent years, with its largest-ever fraud takedown in June 2018 involving over 600 defendants—165 of them medical professionals, including 32 physicians—and costing Medicare and Medicaid over $2 billion. This action, as with many others, involved mass prescription of opioids (Office of the Inspector General, HHS 2018).

In order to systematize these crime-fighting efforts, CMS leadership appointed a new director for its Center for Program Integrity in 2018 and increased the staff responsible for monitoring payments. As of spring 2019, the Center had made some progress in its efforts to leverage government and nongovernmental data sources to detect fraud in the traditional Medicare Program, but it had made less progress on the Medicare Advantage program or on the prescription drug program of Part D (Government Accountability Office 2019a).

A fundamental challenge to payment integrity systems is that CMS has historically operated on a lean staff. This is reflected in Medicare's very low administrative overhead costs, amounting to a mere 1.1 percent in 2017 (Medicare Trustees 2018). This figure is comparable to the figures from recent years. Unlike private insurance companies that hire large numbers of analysts and claims investigators to minimize payments, and frequently spend over 20 percent of their revenue on administrative overhead, Medicare typically pays all claims with minimal scrutiny, so long as they do not look suspicious. CMS's move to increase its staff since 2017 will almost certainly help in fighting fraud.

However, so long as, for example, physicians are allowed to claim variable payments for office visit complexities ranging from ratings of "low," "moderate," or "high" based on factors not directly visible or even verifiable to claims inspectors, Medicare's door for overutilization will remain wide open.

Conclusion

Most of the challenges discussed here have to do with money, and this should not be a surprise, given that the Medicare and Medicaid programs combined account for about 30 percent of the nation's total health care expenditures. They represent a major commitment on the part of taxpayers over a half century to try to meet the needs of vulnerable populations, whether they are children in low-income families, single parents, senior citizens, or the disabled. In keeping with the long tradition in the United States to build social programs of limited scope and that which focus on the needs of discrete categories of individuals, Medicare and Medicaid leave some people either without coverage or without the right kind of coverage. Middle-class Americans account for most of such coverage gaps, particularly those in need of long-term or nursing home care. In light of an aging population, political pressure is likely to grow in the coming years, though expansions of the covered categories will, if history is any indication, be only slowly forthcoming.

Many of the problems and challenges discussed in this chapter disproportionately affect particular groups, some of which are well organized to bring political pressure to bear on policy makers. Hospital associations and nursing home owners are two such examples. Chapter 3 begins to introduce some of these actors, including hospital leaders and lobbying organizations. Other perspectives come from scholars and program users. These perspectives will help readers to dig deeper into the problems and challenges introduced here. The profiles in Chapter 4 will further expand the range of actors involved with these two programs.

Sources

Aaron, Henry, and Jeanne Lambrew. 2008. *Reforming Medicare: Options, Tradeoffs, and Opportunities*. Washington, D.C.: Brookings Institution Press.

Abaluck, Jason, and Jonathan Gruber. 2011. "Choice Inconsistencies Among the Elderly: Evidence from Plan Choice in the Medicare Part D Program." *American Economic Review* 101 (4): 1180–210.

American Hospital Association. 2018. "Uncompensated Hospital Care Cost Fact Sheet" (January).

American Hospital Association. 2019. "AHA Statement on Senate 'Medicare for All' Proposal," press release (April 10).

America's Health Insurance Plans. 2019. "It's Time to Fix the Incorrect Funding Formula for Medicare Advantage Plans," blog post (March 15).

Béland, Daniel, Philip Rocco, and Alex Wadden. 2016. *The Obamacare Wars: Federalism, State Politics, and the Affordable Care Act*. Lawrence: University Press of Kansas.

Blahous, Charles. 2018. The Costs of a National Single-Payer Healthcare System," report from the Mercatus Center, George Mason University (July).

Census Bureau. 2018. Quick Facts data sheet, Washington, D.C. (July).

Center for Medicare Advocacy. 2019. "Analysis of President Trump's Medicare Executive Order" (October 10).

Centers for Medicare and Medicaid Services. 2018. Memo to the Missouri Department of Social Services (November 30). Available at www.medicaid.gov/State-resource-center /Medicaid-State-Plan-Amendments/Downloads/MO/MO -18-0016.pdf (accessed July 8, 2020).

Centers for Medicare and Medicaid Services. 2019. "Comparing Reimbursement Rates," fact sheet on Medicaid rates. Washington, D.C.

Congressional Budget Office. 2013. "A Premium Support System for Medicare: Analysis of Illustrative Options," Washington, D.C. (September).

Congressional Budget Office. 2014. "Competition and the Cost of Medicare's Prescription Drug Program," Washington, D.C. (July).

Congressional Budget Office. 2017. "An Analysis of Hospital Prices for Commercial and Medicare Advantage Plans," Washington, D.C. (June 26).

Congressional Budget Office. 2019. "An Update to the Budget and Economic Outlook: 2019 to 2029," Washington, D.C. (August 21).

Cubanski, Juliette, and Tricia Neuman. 2018. "The Facts on Medicare Spending and Financing," report from the Kaiser Family Foundation (June 22).

Cunningham, Peter, and Ann O'Malley. 2008. "Do Reimbursement Delays Discourage Medicaid Participation by Physicians?" *Health Affairs* 27 (1): w17–18.

Cunningham, Peter, and Jessica May. 2006. "Medicaid Patients Increasingly Concentrated among Physicians," report from the Center for Studying Health System Change (August).

Department of Justice. 2019. "Texas Physician Convicted in $16 Million Medicare Fraud Scheme," press release (October 7).

Duggan, Mark, Amanda Starc, and Boris Vabson. 2016. "Who Benefits When the Government Pays More? Pass-through in the Medicare Advantage Plan." *Journal of Public Economics* 141: 50–67.

Ellison, Alya. 2019. "State-by-State Breakdown of 102 Rural Hospital Closures," report from Beckerhospitalreview.com (March 20).

Enthoven, Alain. 1980. *Health Plan: The Only Practical Solution to the Soaring Cost of Medical Care.* Reading, MA: Addison-Wesley.

Government Accountability Office. 2013a. "Prescription Drugs: Comparison of DOD and VA Direct Purchase Prices," Washington, D.C. (April).

Government Accountability Office. 2013b. "Clinical Data Registries: HHS Could Improve Medicare Quality and Efficiency through Key Requirements and Oversight," Washington, D.C. (December).

Government Accountability Office. 2014. "Medicare: Contractors and Private Plans Play a Major Role in Administering Benefits," Washington, D.C. (March 4).

Government Accountability Office. 2016. "Medicare Advantage: Fundamental Improvements Needed in CMS's Effort to Recover Substantial Amounts of Improper Payments," Washington, D.C. (April).

Government Accountability Office. 2018a. "Medicare: CMS Should Take Actions to Continue Prior Authorization Efforts to Reduce Spending," Washington, D.C. (April).

Government Accountability Office. 2018b. "Medicare: Actions Needed to Better Manage Fraud Risks," Washington, D.C. (July).

Government Accountability Office. 2018c. "Medicaid: Access to Health Care for Low-Income Adults in States with and without Expanded Eligibility," Washington, D.C. (September).

Government Accountability Office. 2019a. "Substantial Efforts Needed to Achieve Greater Progress on High-Risk Areas," Washington, D.C. (March 6).

Government Accountability Office. 2019b. "Health: Prior Authorization in Medicare," Washington, D.C. (March 29).

Hayes, Susan, Akeissa Coleman, Sara Collins, and Rachel Nuzam. 2019. "The Fiscal Case for Medicaid Expansion," report from the Commonwealth Fund (February 15).

Healy, Jack. 2019. "Nursing Homes Are Closing across Rural America, Scattering Residents," *New York Times* (March 14).

Herzlinger, Regina. 1997. *Market Driven Health Care: Who Wins, Who Loses in the Transformation of America's Largest Service Industry*. Cambridge, MA: Perseus Books.

Holahan, John, Linda Blumberg, Lisa Clemans-Cope, Siyabonga Ndwandwe, Matthew Buettgens, and Melissa Favreault. 2016. "The Sanders Single-Payer Health Care Plan," report from the Urban Institute (May).

Holgash, Kayla, and Martha Heberlein. 2019. "Physician Acceptance of New Medicaid Patients: What Matters and What Doesn't," Health Affairs Blog (April 10).

Jacobson, Gretchen, Anthony Damico, and Tricia Neuman. 2018. "A Dozen Facts about Medicare Advantage," report from the Kaiser Family Foundation (November).

Jacobson, Gretchen, and Tricia Neuman. 2016. "Turning Medicare into a Premium Support System: Frequently Asked Questions," report from the Kaiser Family Foundation (July).

Johnson, Akilah. 2019. "Medicare for All Is Not Medicare, and Not Really for All. So What Does It Actually Mean?" ProPublica (September 16).

Johnson, James, Carleen Stoskopf, and Leiyu Shi. 2018. *Comparative Health Systems: A Global Perspective, 2nd edition*. Burlington, MA: Jones and Bartlett Learning.

Jost, Timothy. 2007. *Health Care at Risk: A Critique of the Consumer-Driven Movement*. Durham, NC: Duke University Press.

Kaiser Family Foundation. 2019a. "The Coverage Gap: Uninsured Poor Adults in States That Do Not Expand Medicaid" (March 21).

Kaiser Family Foundation. 2019b. July Health Tracking Poll.

Keith, Katie, and Timothy Jost. 2017. "Unpacking the Sanders Medicare-For-All Bill," a blog from *Health Affairs* (September 14).

Kronick, Richard. 2017. "Projected Coding Intensity in Medicare Advantage Could Increase Medicare Spending by $200 Billion over Ten Years," *Health Affairs* 26 (2, February).

LaMattina, John. 2016. "Gilead's CEO Admits to 'Failures' in Setting Price of $1,000-A-Pill Breakthrough," *Forbes* (December 8).

Liberman, Liz. 2018. "Medicaid Reimbursement Rates Draw Attention," report from the National Investment Center for Seniors Housing & Care (March 21).

Marmor, Theodore. 2003. "Evolution of the American Social Contract for Care," in David Blumenthal, Marilyn Moon, Mark Warshawsky, and Cristina Boccuti (eds.), *Long-Term Care and Medicare Policy: Can We Improve the Continuity of Care?* Washington, D.C.: National Academy of Social Insurance.

Medicaid and CHIP Payment Access Commission. 2019. "Disproportionate Share Hospital Payments," Washington, D.C.

Medicare Payment Advisory Commission. 2018. "Medicare Payment Policy," Washington, D.C. (March).

Medicare Trustees. 2018. Annual Report of the Boards of Trustees of the Federal Hospital Insurance and Federal Supplemental Medical Insurance Trust Funds. Washington, D.C. (June).

Medicare Trustees. 2019. Annual Report of the Boards of Trustees of the Federal Hospital Insurance and Federal Supplemental Medical Insurance Trust Funds. Washington, D.C. (April).

Mosley, David, and Daniel DeBehnke. 2019. "Rural Hospital Sustainability: New Analysis Shows Worsening Situation for Rural Hospitals, Residents," report from Navigant (February).

National Committee to Preserve Social Security and Medicare. 2018. "The House Fiscal Year 2019 Budget and Its Effect on Seniors" (June 29).

Neuman, Tricia, and Gretchen Jacobson. 2017. "Medicare Premium Support Proposals Could Increase Costs for Today's Seniors, Despite Assurances," *Health Affairs Blog* (March 9).

Neuman, Tricia, and Gretchen Jacobson. 2018. "Medicare Advantage Checkup." *The New England Journal of Medicine* 379 (22): 2,163–172.

Oberlander, Jonathan. 2003. *The Political Life of Medicare.* Chicago: University of Chicago Press.

Office of the Inspector General, Department of Health and Human Services. 2018. "2018 National Health Care Fraud Takedown," press release (June).

Oliver, Thomas, Philip Lee, and Helene Lipton. 2004. "A Political History of Medicare and Prescription Drug Coverage." *The Milbank Quarterly* 82 (2): 283–354.

Papanicolas, Irene, Liana Woskie, and Ashish Jha. 2018. "Health Care Spending in the United States and Other High-Income Countries." *The Journal of the American Medical Association* 319 (10):1024–39.

Paradise, Julia. 2017. "Data Note: A Large Majority of Physicians Participate in Medicaid," report from the Kaiser Family Foundation (May).

Parkins, Katie. 2018. "Seniors Look to Lawmakers to Bridge Gap in Missouri Medicaid Funding," *Missourian* newspaper (March 13).

Pharmaceutical Research and Manufacturers of America. 2019. "PhRMA Statement Opposing Senate Finance Committee Drug Pricing Legislation," press release (September 13).

Potetz, Lisa, Juliette Cubanski, and Tricia Neuman. 2011. "Medicare Spending and Financing: A Primer," report from the Kaiser Family Foundation (February).

Potter, Wendell, and Nick Penniman. 2016. *Nation on the Take: How Big Money Corrupts Our Democracy and What We Can Do about It*. New York: Bloomsbury Press.

Quadagno, Jill. 2015. "The Transformation of Medicaid from Poor Law Legacy to Middle-Class Entitlement," in Alan Cohen, David Colby, Keith Wailoo, and Julian Zelizer (eds.). *Medicare and Medicaid at 50: America's Entitlement Programs in the Age of Affordable Care*. New York: Oxford University Press.

Ramsey, Lydia. 2019. "How Much a Nursing Home Room Costs in All 50 States," Businessinsider.com (March 4).

Shaw, Greg M. 2017. *The Dysfunctional Politics of the Affordable Care Act*. Santa Barbara, CA: Praeger Publishers.

Shih, Chuck, Jordan Schwartz, and Allan Coukell. 2016. "How Would Government Negotiation of Medicare Part D Drug Prices Work?" *Health Affairs Blog* (February 1).

Smedley, Brian, Adrienne Stith, and Alan Nelson, eds. 2003. *Unequal Treatment: Confronting Racial and Ethnic Disparities in Healthcare*. Washington, D.C.: National Academies Press.

Woolhandler, Steffie, and David Himmelstiein. 2017. "Single-Payer Reform: The Only Way to Fulfill the President's Pledge of More Coverage, Better Benefits, and Lower Costs." *Annals of Internal Medicine* 166 (8): 587–88.

Zarabozo, Carlos. 2000. "Milestone in Medicare Managed Care." *Health Care Financing Review* 22 (1): 61–67.

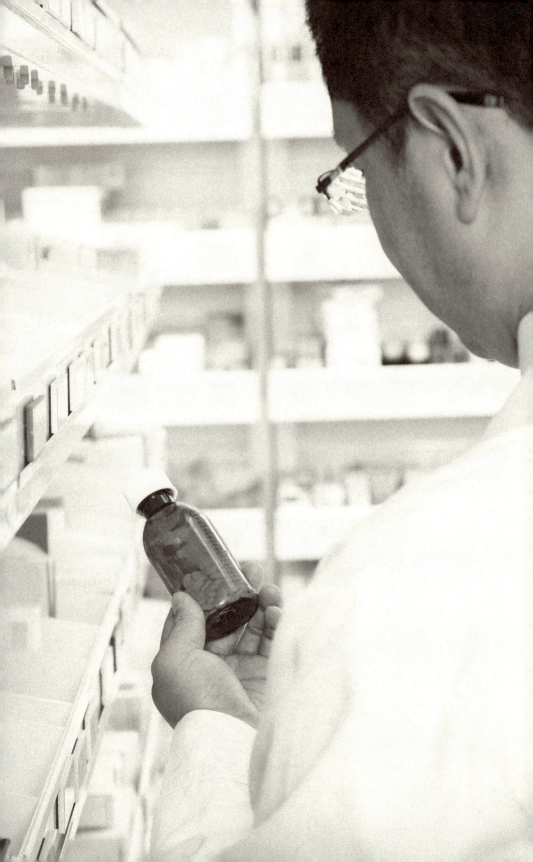

Medicare and Medicaid's half-century of history has been imprinted deeply into Americans' ways of thinking about health care provision and financing. These programs steer providers to deliver certain kinds of treatments rather than others. They have convinced many Americans that health care is, or at least should be, a basic citizenship right. Together they have established a massive footprint in the annual federal budget, accounting for approximately 25 percent of it in recent years. Almost no one calls for their abolition, and few people call for significant retrenchment in these areas. But providers, patients, and taxpayers also recognize major shortcomings in both Medicare and Medicaid. Of the many things that can be said about these programs, two chief complaints are that they do not cover enough people or a broad enough range of services as many participants would like and that neither program pays providers enough to ensure ready access by beneficiaries to all of the caregivers they want to see.

This chapter consists of nine essays contributed by medical providers, program beneficiaries, policy advocates, and scholars. The providers represent both small and large organizations, both for-profit and not-for-profit. Contributors' essays speak to their personal experiences and their organizations' efforts to

A pharmacist reviews the label on a prescription drug bottle. Americans spent $335 billion on prescription drugs in 2018. (Shannon Fagan/Dreamstime.com)

help those in need. However, these persons are also cognizant of the strengths and the very real limitations of Medicare and Medicaid. These organizations have shown a good deal of flexibility and creativity in meshing Medicaid in particular with the realities of running expensive clinical operations. Considering these programs from users' perspectives, a pair of essays from beneficiaries tell of not only the usefulness of government insurance but also the challenges of applying this coverage in some situations. The contributions from policy scholars help situate the programs and some of the controversies discussed in Chapter 2 in the larger political context that prevails these days. Specifically, there is a broad sense that government assistance should do more to help those persons in need, particularly to address the grave inequalities in both service access and health outcomes across social groups. However, so long as other political actors resent the high costs of these programs, federal and state governments are unlikely to fund Medicare and Medicaid at the levels that universal and high-quality access would require. Some of this political context is directly attributable to lingering partisan resentment over Obamacare, and some of it has to do with the broader, decades-long debate about the proper role of government in Americans' lives more fundamentally.

As complicated and far-reaching as Medicare and Medicaid are, they cannot be portrayed in a single snapshot; rather, describing them requires more of a mosaic or a series of perspectives. The programs are many things to many people. Together, these essays take another step toward portraying them in all of their complexity. The opinions voiced by these contributors are their own.

My Journey on Medicaid
Aianna Zachary

As a single mother of two and someone who lives with chronic health challenges, Medicaid has been of great value in my life.

It paid for my children's births. It has given me a sense of security as I have sought complicated medical treatments for my kids, one who has severe asthma. It covers some of the prescriptions for my two sons and me. Given all of the challenges in my life, Medicaid has allowed me to worry a little less about my family's health, even though the way the program works with doctors and clinics has not always been perfect.

I first went on to Medicaid at age 19 in Oklahoma when I became pregnant with my first son. The application was easy, and the program served me well so long as I was carrying a child. I could seek treatment anytime I needed anything, even if it was related to my overall health versus the pregnancy. They would check me out. I didn't have to worry. However, upon my son's birth, Medicaid in Oklahoma ended my eligibility, since it was really designed to cover his needs and not mine. I found myself without health insurance. When, due to a health problem, I needed to get my thyroid levels checked but didn't have any way to pay for that, I went back into the public assistance office. My husband and I didn't have any money. We were living hand to mouth. I was scared and sick, and I was denied coverage. The social worker said, "Have another baby." That was sincere advice from them, but I was angry and sad. I didn't want to have another baby just to be able to go see the doctor. It didn't seem like a very good solution, to say the least. So, I got help from family, which is what you do in that situation. That sort of got me through for a while.

I spent several years uninsured, skipping the care that I needed due to my autoimmune disease. My husband's way of moving in and out of jobs meant we had insurance sometimes but no coverage at other times. We tried to use COBRA coverage, but that was usually too expensive. That increased the amount of time we had to wait for coverage of preexisting conditions. A second child eventually came along, and his medicines were about $800 per month at the time. Selling jewelry helped raise a little money for visits to doctors. You do what you have to do. For the kids, Oklahoma was willing to cover them up to age five under its SoonerCare program, but this left me without coverage.

Finally, in 2016, after a divorce, I decided to move to Illinois. I wanted to go back to school. I was working and doing really well at that. But health care has been something that always gave me a lot of anxiety and stress. My sister had moved there the year before, and knowing that my kids and I could get basic care and always have a place to go meant the move made sense for us. I knew that Illinois had expanded its Medicaid program, and that was very, very attractive. Oklahoma did not. The application in Illinois was very easy. I went to the office downtown. I filled out the paperwork and had an interview, and the determination of our eligibility was all very straightforward. Within a couple of weeks, my kids and I had health insurance. This came as a great relief. In addition to covering office visits, Illinois's Medicaid program also helps with most of the prescriptions my family needs. The recertification of my eligibility every six months is usually routine, and even when some paperwork fell between the cracks, my social worker renewed my eligibility back to the previous period of coverage. The process of getting coverage has been very smooth.

While I'm happy to have the insurance coverage, using it is sometimes challenging. I'm settled into my coverage, but I'm not always happy with it. I found a nonprofit clinic, and the doctor there is very, very good at her job. But she and some of the other staff there are busy, so we're not getting good enough access to appointments. A lot of those visits just aren't happening right now. I know that not going is not a solution, but it's just not happening right now. Beyond this clinic, lots of other doctors won't accept Medicaid, and this is particularly true for specialists. My son's asthma means he needs to find a pediatric pulmonologist. These are few and far between as it is, and to find one locally who will accept Medicaid has proven nearly impossible. Traveling to distant communities to visit one is hard, given unreliable personal transportation. We have missed a lot of appointments, and this only makes my son's struggle with asthma at school even harder. Our Medicaid-managed care plan also makes it hard to find all the providers we need. Some don't accept our particular plan, even if they accept Medicaid generally.

Another problem has been prescription drug coverage. I'm happy that Illinois covers most of what I need and doesn't limit me to three scripts per month like Oklahoma did, and I'm happy that I can find pharmacies that are willing to accept my insurance. But because of an emerging condition similar to fibromyalgia, I would benefit from a drug that the Medicaid plan doesn't cover. So I can't get it.

Choice is really important to me. People are individuals, and what I really miss is not just general availability but being able to find someone you can connect with, who will listen to you, and who is actually going to help you get better. That can be hard under the best of circumstances. When I started getting really sick, finding a doctor who took me seriously was really hard. As a person living with a chronic disease, I need to see doctors more often than most. I have found out that it's very, very common for a woman in my circumstances to be treated like I'm being hysterical. Part of finding health care means having options. That's what's most limiting to me: not having options. Right now, I can go to this clinic, but even there I still have to be my own advocate. It's hard to know if the clinic's resources, stretched as thinly as they are, are to blame, but I'm not entirely satisfied with things there. It's important to note that my doctors have been very supportive on the financial side. But as a person on Medicaid, I'm aware that my options are so limited, so I have to make choices, hard trade-offs. The whole thing feels like a concession, and it feels like a concession on something that I know is only going to get worse. And so it's very, very stressful. But I'm grateful to have something.

Aianna Zachary is an artist and single mother of two. She lives and works in central Illinois. She and her children have benefited from Medicaid on and off over many years while living in Oklahoma and Illinois.

Medicaid and the Family Medicine Practice
Adam Houghton, MD

I don't care about your insurance. I really don't. When you are sitting across from me in the exam room, your insurance is one of the last things on my mind. But your insurance plan won't let me ignore them for too long. In fact, modern medical insurance plans have a tendency to jump up and down and play doctor. That blood test I want to order isn't covered. That medication I want to prescribe you is not preferred on your formulary. That MRI I want to run needs a prior authorization. Good luck meeting your ridiculously high deductible. But worst of all, your insurance plan may make it harder and harder for me to see you at all. I am happy to see anyone regardless of their age, race, gender identity, sexual orientation, political leanings, creed, or musical preference. So what could possibly be the reason that I may have to turn you away? It boils down to that thing we don't like to openly talk about in medicine: money. When I talk about profits made from office visits or procedures, I feel that it makes our work sound greedy and selfish. I did not choose this career path in order to make a buck. How do I reconcile the altruistic practice of medicine with the stark truth of the business of medicine? How can I live in that world and still make a difference?

The financial realities of various insurance plans, while frustrating, are something that any medical practice, especially a small, independent practice, cannot ignore. Since Medicaid is funded both by the federal government and states, the percentage of reimbursement compared to Medicare varies state by state. A common way to analyze reimbursement patterns is based on a percentage of Medicare reimbursement. At the time this piece was written, the reimbursement for Medicaid in my state was around 70 percent of what Medicare would pay for the same service. Now, this is an overall average, which can still vary quite a bit among various medical codes. Commercial insurance plans generally pay 115–130 percent of Medicare rates if not higher. These are not the actual charges, but the easy math is that if I provide a service, let's say an office visit to manage your high blood pressure and diabetes, and Medicare will reimburse $100 for that office visit, a Medicaid plan would pay about $70 for that same service, while a commercial plan may pay $130 or more. In-office ancillary services can show even greater disparities. For example, certain commercial insurance plans consistently pay over double what Medicare pays for in-office ultrasound, whether it is for thyroid, complete abdomen, or veins checking for blood clots. Spread out over thousands of patients and thousands of office visits per year, a practice with a large percentage of Medicare and Medicaid plans will be reimbursed dramatically less for the same services compared to a practice with a larger percentage of commercial insurance plans. A large hospital system can offset costs through subsidizing areas of financial loss with gains they may make elsewhere. However, a small medical practice generally has to limit the number of Medicaid or Medicare patients it sees in order to stay afloat.

A separate payment issue revolves around accounts receivable, which is the amount that the insurance companies have not yet paid. If I see you in the office today, complete my office note, and submit the charges to your insurance, your insurance company does not pay me immediately. Medicare plans generally pay within two to three weeks, which seems pretty reasonable. Medicaid in our practice in Illinois currently is out around 120 days. At one point, Medicaid accounts receivable were as far as 300 days out. So when I see a patient with a Medicaid plan, not only will the payment for an office visit be about 30 percent less than Medicare and almost as little as half what a high reimbursing commercial plan would be, but also I may not receive that payment for a number of months.

Any medical practice and medical building also has overhead. We pay providers, staff salaries, and benefits. We pay our internet and phone bills. We pay our rent or mortgage. We pay for office supplies and toilet paper. By calculating out an office overhead each month and the number of visits each month, we can get an idea of the average reimbursement per office visit needed to cover the operating costs of the office. With Medicaid, the payment rates for an office visit are below the overhead cost of providing care for that office visit. So not only will the payment be 30 percent less than Medicare and almost half of what a commercial plan might pay three to four months later than other payments, but also the office will effectively lose money on that office visit since the amount paid will not cover the overhead costs for the visit.

While there are a variety of Medicaid programs for each state, those who qualify for Medicaid in all states include some low-income individuals, families, and children as well as pregnant women, the elderly, and people with disabilities. Medicaid covers all low-income adults below a certain income level in some states. These populations often have difficulty accessing other health care services, such as dental and vision care. Low-income populations may also have further social needs than those with more resources. Transportation issues can lead to higher office visit no-show rates, especially during harsh weather seasons or inclement conditions. These individuals also may have difficulty affording prescribed medications. With these traditional limitations to health care access, these patients may also have more advanced disease processes, such as diabetes, high blood pressure, and heart disease. It can be difficult for primary care offices to find specialty groups that will accept Medicaid plans, so I may end up treating more complex disease states without the assistance of other specialists. Poorly covered services also can lead to crippling debt, especially under dual-eligible patients with Medicare and Medicaid. Since Medicaid pays around 70 percent and Medicare covers 80 percent for Part B charges, the patient can be on the hook for the 20 percent remainder of the bill, which would generally be picked up if they had a different supplemental plan. Medical bills are the number one cause of bankruptcy in the United States. I did not go into medicine to bankrupt my patients. So now we are getting reimbursed less to the point where the office loses money on that office visit, we are not receiving the portion of reimbursement to offset some overhead costs for a number of months, we are spending more time per visit managing complex health and social-emotional issues, and oh, by the way, patients are getting slammed with unpaid medical bills. My repetition here is purposeful in order to drive home the point that smaller, independent practices cannot see large numbers of patients with Medicaid plans and stay in business. And a major priority of a business is to stay in business. So the question remains: What are we to do to still help everyone in our community? Where do we even start?

As a primary care provider, I despise the idea of limiting the number of patients I can see based on their specific insurance plan or life situation. I did not become a doctor in order to only think about the bottom line or to disparage someone with a less favorable insurance plan. I do see patients with Medicaid plans, but we do limit the number that we are able to accept. So what are the alternatives? An excellent model available is a Federally Qualified Health Center (FQHC). These medical practices must meet several standards in order to qualify, and they are meant to provide care for underserved communities. An FQHC charges a flat fee per visit rather than separate charges for different levels of office visits and ancillary charges, such as a flu swab or strep swab. Patients may also have much lower co-pays at an FQHC compared to an independent or hospital-based practice. An FQHC can collect higher reimbursements due to the fact that, as implied by their name, they are funded through the federal, rather than state, government. These payments are also received in a few weeks. Hospital, university, or large group affiliated practices have more ability to provide access due to sheer volume and deeper pockets to offset cost. Residency programs, which are training programs for physicians affiliated with a university or hospital, traditionally see a large underserved population. These types of medical practices are not available in every community, but they are a tremendous benefit where available. I have completed a residency program, and I have worked at a FQHC. We should be encouraging and helping establish these models. I am lucky enough to have all of these options in my community. So even if there are groups of people I am not able to see in large volumes based on their insurance carrier, I can help navigate those patients to our local FQHC, residency program, or hospital-based practices. Medicine is a team effort. We can partner with other health care providers or align ourselves with larger entities in order to better serve our populations. Maybe I won't be able to take you on as a patient here, but at least I can guide you to someone who can. And barring radical changes in the way of insurance and medical reimbursement, I may have to learn to live with that. I really don't care about your insurance. But I really do care about doing the best that I can with the resources I have available. I think that's a start.

Adam Houghton, MD, is a board-certified family medicine physician and part-owner of Bloomington Primary Care, an independent family medicine practice in Bloomington, Illinois. He completed medical school at Southern Illinois University School of Medicine and his residency training at Memorial Hospital in South Bend, Indiana.

A Nonprofit Clinic's Perspective on Medicare and Medicaid
Tory Lynch-Dahmm

Most of us identify basic human needs as including not only food and shelter but also sanitation, education, and health care. In the United States, obtaining the basic need of health care becomes quite a challenge without insurance, especially for those with a lower income or no income at all. For most people, private health insurance is obtained through their employer or a family member's employer or is purchased by the individual for themselves and their families. However, individuals without an employer who provides or those facing other financial constraints cannot afford private insurance. For this population, a public option for health care, Medicaid or Medicare, is the better option rather than go without insurance.

Health care providers deemed as Federally Qualified Health Centers (FQHCs) provide services to a population that is uninsured, underinsured, or covered through Medicare, Medicaid, or other state insurance vendors. While some private health care providers shy away from accepting patients with publicly funded insurance due to the low reimbursement rate, FQHCs will accept public payers because they receive an enhanced Medicaid and Medicare rate that is not based on the typical Evaluation and Management coding practices in which services coded as more complex are reimbursed at a higher level. Instead, the enhanced Medicaid and Medicare rate is determined based on the organization's actual costs.

FQHC organizations may also receive additional funding from the federal Health Resources and Service Administration, a part of the U.S. Department of Health and Human Services, to assist in operating their health center. With additional funding, FQHCs are able to provide an enhanced service experience for their patients, which can include case management, patient education, transportation, outreach, and community health workers. FQHC organizations welcome individuals with Medicare or Medicaid and encourage noninsured patients to obtain the benefit of Medicaid if they qualify.

Individuals who have not had insurance due to their financial constraints may neglect their health and seek services only when their medical conditions become significant challenges in their lives. By then, the medical services they seek would often become costlier, especially when the services are obtained through an emergency department instead of through a traditional outpatient provider's office. The patchwork coverage that often results from being uninsured set up many individuals for problems that more consistent care could avoid. In contrast, those individuals who do have Medicare and Medicaid coverage are able to obtain routine medical care for acute and chronic conditions as well as preventative medical services. Research has demonstrated that preventative medicine can reduce the future costs of medical care for some individuals and prevent some chronic conditions.

FQHCs have seen transformative experiences in our patients when they have access to quality medical services. Individuals who experienced chronic conditions often report feeling isolated and depressed. However, with regular health care, these individuals improve not only their health but also the quality of their life and their personal relationships.

One such experience occurred with one of our patients. Barry, 64 years old, had been homeless most of his adult life, living in various shelters and moving to warmer or cooler areas throughout the year. As a result of Barry's living situation, which included a poor diet with few vegetables and fruits, he developed diabetes and hypertension. His chronic conditions were causing dangerous consequences to his health. At one point, it was unsafe for Barry to live in the shelter because he could not routinely access critically needed services. With the help of the FQHC case managers, Barry was able to get care in a long-term nursing facility. During his stay there, his chronic conditions were managed with medications and diet. Upon discharge from the long-term care facility, the FQHC case managers assisted Barry in finding housing specifically for older individuals with a low income. For the past four years, Barry has been living independently, maintaining his health through regular visits with his primary care provider. Barry reduced the number of times he frequented the emergency department from monthly to one to two times a year (for actual emergencies). This transformation would not have been possible without public insurance.

Medicaid also assists families who otherwise would lack insurance. Low-income families whose adult members are unemployed, or who are employed but do not have insurance for all members of the family, are also able to obtain medical care for their entire family at an FQHC. In most cases, the children of the family will qualify for Medicaid. Research has shown that children without routine quality health care are more likely to have higher absenteeism from school and lower grades. For most children, preventative or well-child visits are the only medical care necessary outside of a few visits a year for acute medical conditions, such as strep throat or injuries. However, families without insurance are likely to forego preventative visits due to the cost, which can cost anywhere from $100 for the office visit to up to $500 for vaccinations. This can result in the child falling behind on her or his vaccination schedule. It can also result in missed opportunities to intervene with developmental concerns that are evaluated during well-child visits. The Early and Periodic Screening, Diagnostic, and Treatment components of Medicaid were designed to ensure this important coverage for children, but, of course, it is only available to those who are enrolled in this public insurance program.

Medicaid was instrumental in providing help to a single mother of three named Mandy when her youngest child was born with a genetic condition that impacted his eyesight, hearing, and developmental growth. Without the public medical insurance, her son would not have had access to the numerous specialty providers who regularly follow his care and prescribe daily medication, the Cochlear ear implant that has aided his hearing, or the various speech and physical therapists who have worked with him since birth to address his condition. With Medicaid coverage, the quality of life for this child improved dramatically.

Publicly funded insurances such as Medicare and Medicare provide an opportunity for those with a lower income to have access to quality health care services. FQHC organizations recognize the value of publicly funded health insurance for the individuals and families served. While there are challenges for providers who accept Medicare and Medicaid in terms of getting certain medical tests and procedures covered by these programs, the benefits far outweigh the challenges when the health of our patients is transformed.

Tory Lynch-Dahmm has been employed by Chestnut Health Systems, a nonprofit health care organization, for over 30 years. Since 1973, Chestnut Health Systems has provided behavioral health services. In 2012, the organization evolved its service line to include primary care services and became designated as a Federally Qualified Health Center. She has a master's degree in counseling psychology and a master's in business administration from Illinois State University. She manages the health center's quality improvement program and grant reporting. In addition, she is the co-administrator for the health center's electronic medical record system.

Closing the Gap in Health Care Access
Amanda F. Hopkins, PhD, RN

When nurses are working with patients who receive Medicaid, it's not uncommon to hear various people engage in remarks that are judgmental: "Well, they've got Medicaid, so why don't they take better care of their health?" Negative comments of this nature are judgmental, demonstrate closed-mindedness, perpetuate harmful stereotypes, and are detrimental to building open communication and trust in patient-provider relationships. Many people, including health care providers, struggle with preconceived notions when encountering individuals on Medicaid, and they often assume that Medicaid coverage ensures equal opportunity and access to safe and reliable care. In addition to dispelling common myths surrounding "Medicaid patients," nurses have a powerful platform for sharing observations and experiences of how vulnerable and underrepresented populations attempt to navigate the health care system in a world where they are often invisible. Throughout history, nurses have listened to and addressed the concerns of those whose voices go unheard by using innovative and creative methods to respond to changes in the regulation and financing of health care. Nurses have a professional responsibility to raise awareness of disparities and of barriers that facilitate disparities and to encourage action toward closing the health care gaps.

Disparities based on the intersectionality of race, ethnicity, sexuality, and socioeconomic status continue to be challenges in the United States, where health care is an often overlooked area of division. Throughout history, infectious disease outbreaks have affected society's most vulnerable and underrepresented populations. We need to look no further than the current COVID-19 global pandemic, where the colored people and immigrants in United States are affected by the virus at disproportionate rates compared to white citizens, to see evidence of history repeating itself. Consequently, these disparities persist regarding access to quality and affordable health care. The U.S. Department of Health and Human Services characterizes underrepresented, underserved, and vulnerable populations as communities that include people with low incomes, members of minority populations, and/or individuals who have experienced health disparities. Because they are less likely to have health insurance due to the high costs, many have little interaction with providers, often since childhood, resulting in an overall lack of knowledge about how to navigate these systems. On average, vulnerable groups experience restricted health care access, lower quality of care, and markedly poorer health outcomes compared to other U.S. populations. Further, they experience twice the number of behavioral health problems and are commonly socially isolated. The fact that underrepresented, underserved, and vulnerable populations are the least healthy groups in the United States, or that Black Americans are dying from COVID-19 at higher rates than any other group, is not due to chance. It is well documented that the institutional and systematic effects of racism may be the most important concept underlying health disparities of vulnerable populations. And while the Medicaid program and its expansion over the past several years has led to significant improvements in access to care and health outcomes for vulnerable and underrepresented populations, challenges persist, and opportunities for further improvement must be examined.

A commonly forgotten population who are from disproportionately low socioeconomic backgrounds and are vulnerable to
poor health outcomes are the imprisoned. The negative impact
of incarceration on health is overwhelming, in large part due to
gaps in access to medical services and prescription medications.
And yet a federal law exists (the Medicaid Inmate Exclusion
Policy), which forces Medicaid-covered inmates, including
those who are jailed but cannot afford bail while awaiting trial,
to lose their health insurance. Although the 2.3 million people
incarcerated in the United States still have a legal right to health
services, their lack of adequate care has been well documented.
As we're currently witnessing with COVID-19, due to the
well-established overcrowding patterns in many jail systems,
infectious diseases spread quickly. Further, many inmates suffer
from mental health issues, and their infectious and chronic disease rates are exponentially higher than their non-incarcerated
counterparts. Upon release, the vast majority of inmates will
return to their previous communities along with their health
conditions, often aggravated by their time in prison, and many
will not have health insurance coverage.

After non-Hispanic Whites and Hispanics, Blacks currently
comprise the third-largest racial or ethnic group in the United
States. As of 2019, 47.4 million (approximately 13%) of individuals living in the United States identified as Black or African
American. Hispanic and Black/African American populations are more likely to be uninsured than Whites, and they
report an inability to seek health care due to cost. In seeking
resolutions to decreasing health care disparities, it is essential
to examine race, as well as financial and nonfinancial barriers, to access health services. The health care system is lacking for many vulnerable and underrepresented populations,
but none so much as for Black Americans. Black Americans
have a higher risk than Whites for health conditions including maternal mortality, infant mortality, heart disease, diabetes,
hypertension, and other health issues. Further, out-of-pocket
costs are often burdensome and a barrier to the health security

of Black Americans. And yet, lack of insurance in Black Americans continues to be a strong predictor of increased mortality. Vision, dental, and mental health Medicaid coverage varies by state, and even if individuals have existing health care coverage, that doesn't guarantee continuity of coverage. With the categorical eligibility of Medicaid beneficiaries changing due to income changes, many cycle on and off the program, creating gaps in coverage.

The issues related to accessing health care are numerous, and access and quality of care in Medicaid programs have never been optimal. Providers are less likely to accept Medicaid patients than people on other types of health care insurance. Many providers indicate lower (and slower) rates of reimbursement to be the primary reason for rejection of these patients. Even if people are able to identify a provider who accepts Medicaid, it doesn't necessarily mean they will be able to secure one of the limited appointments available or have a way to get there. Transportation is an often identified barrier to health care access for individuals living in poor communities. Black Americans are more likely to lack access to hospitals and other health care providers (HCPs) due to residential segregation. Further, health care agencies that treat large populations of minorities tend to face greater challenges in providing high-quality care. Patients who seek HCPs located within predominantly Black American neighborhoods tend to have a lack of trust in HCPs, report lower-quality care, and experience racial bias and stereotyping by providers. Trust facilitates open communication, which is foundational to positive rapport building with patients and their families. Unfortunately, the existing patchwork system of communication hinders patients' ability to form stable and trusting relationships with HCPs. Underrepresented groups are more likely to seek care from HCPs of their own race, ethnicity, and/or culture. Medicaid and Medicare have played a significant role for Black Americans in reducing discrimination including enabling access to medical care. By withholding federal funding from health care agencies that practiced racial discrimination in the 1960s, Medicare forced hospitals to desegregate. The historical impact of health care agencies' discrimination against Black American nurses and doctors (by refusing to hire them) is long lasting and is correlated with the current lack of minority HCPs.

Even if people happen to have transportation to a quality health care institution where trusted providers are employed, there's no guarantee they will be accepted as a patient. As a result, it is not uncommon for these individuals to rely heavily on community health centers and emergency departments when seeking care. Lack of transportation greatly hinders the ability to access all health care services, especially preventive care, which often forces individuals to seek health care only in emergent situations. Emergency department visits are often accessed not by choice, but by lack of other available options. The continued lack of access and lack of a relationship with a primary HCP who accepts Medicaid, accompanied by reduced health care literacy, all contribute to increased misuse of the emergency department.

The historical and current racial discrimination that underrepresented and vulnerable groups continue to suffer clearly underlies their higher than average risk of poor health outcomes. We need look no further than the current COVID-19 crisis to see how existing disparities in health and access to health care in the United States are consequently impacting marginalized communities at disproportionate rates. It's clear that Medicare and Medicaid are vital to the health care needs of many, yet coverage alone is not a guarantee of access for vulnerable communities. The changing demographics in the U.S. population will only result in an increase in diversity, emphasizing the importance for Medicaid as one more mode of meeting the needs of the populations it serves. Necessary improvements must be made to ensure equitable health care for all.

Although Medicaid provision is a great starting point to address the concerns that plague vulnerable and underrepresented populations, Medicaid alone will not resolve all U.S.

health care disparities. In short, to assure health care of the highest quality, and to that of life comparable to other Americans, proactive efforts must be taken to eliminate conscious and unconscious biases impacting health care. An equitable health care system needs to be part of the solution to overcome the many historic burdens that underrepresented groups, especially Black Americans, still bear in the United States. Focused efforts must be directed at all health care systems and providers. Commonly, the vulnerable and underrepresented communities are not invited to the table where strategies and programs addressing their poor health care situations are designed and prioritized. Moreover, many (primarily White) HCPs charged with developing the aforementioned strategies and programs have very little to no experience with, or understanding of, the cultural or historical context of these groups. How are members of vulnerable and underrepresented communities supposed to trust that a true commitment to increasing their positive health care outcomes exists, or that the developed interventions will be effective, when they are developed by those with limited knowledge of them as a group? It is well documented that cultural awareness (of self and others) coupled with education may be the most important tools HCPs have to change the operation of current systems. Mandatory training in cultural sensitivity and in self-awareness of unconscious biases, along with regular recertification, should be implemented in all health care systems. We must make it our responsibility to translate our health care knowledge into the language and culture of the specific clients we serve. Additionally, the demographics of health care professionals needs to reflect that of those communities they serve. Further research and action are needed to identify and implement solutions so that all Americans are afforded the same health care opportunities.

Amanda F. Hopkins is an Associate Professor in the School of Nursing at Illinois Wesleyan University. Dr. Hopkins earned a BSN from the University of Illinois at Chicago, where she later received her MS and PhD. As a pediatric nurse and educator, Dr. Hopkins has expertise in working with underrepresented and vulnerable populations, including children with chronic conditions and their families. Dr. Hopkins's research focuses on the study of providing culturally competent, family-centered care in addition to creating culturally competent health care work environments.

Medicaid and Emergency Department Use
Mollie Ward, MDiv

Medicaid patients are sometimes forced to make what can seem like myopic choices about their health care, and their all too frequent use of hospital emergency departments for non-emergent conditions is one unfortunate outcome of this dynamic. As U.S. hospitals have come under increasing pressure to make do with less, they have scrambled to find the ways to optimize the use of their resources. In this climate, data showing use of emergency departments for non-emergent issues are eye-catching, especially when fully 50 percent of non-emergent ED cases in one Midwestern hospital in recent years were Medicaid patients originating in specific areas of the community. Hospitals consider ED usage for the treatment of non-emergent cases problematic for several reasons. From a financial perspective, EDs are the most expensive place for patients to receive care because of the specialties and technology required to effectively run and equip a modern emergency department, and because it costs more, many insurance plans charge significant co-pays for non-emergent use of EDs. Moreover, despite our best efforts, from a coordination of care perspective, inappropriate use of EDs tends to lead to episodic, crisis-oriented care rather than an approach based on long-term relationships and the kind of big-picture planning that provides the best health outcomes. The hard reality facing many Medicaid beneficiaries is that some one-third of doctors in the average community either do not accept Medicaid as payment or they severely limit the number of such patients they will treat. This leads to an access problem that in turn leads these persons to the doors of their local ED, even though better options exist. Based on the experience of the hospital where my colleagues and I work, there are ways for institutions and communities to work together to steer patients in beneficial directions that can broaden the care options for patients as well as benefit other stakeholders.

Some of these innovative directions were recently pursued by the Central Illinois community of Bloomington-Normal, where in 2016 an interdisciplinary taskforce sought to discover the reasons so many Medicaid patients living in certain "hot zones" were using Carle BroMenn Medical Center's ED for routine health care. As part of this taskforce, hospital chaplains worked with our Delegate Church Association, a group of 80-plus faith communities that supports the hospital's health care ministry, to gather information from Medicaid patients about their ED use. The study, based on 28 in-depth interviews was small, but the findings were both reassuring and daunting.

The findings were reassuring because some were initially concerned that perhaps Medicaid patients were unaware of what is an inappropriate use of the ED. But most of those interviewed—the majority of whom were Medicaid patients who had used the ED in the previous two years—easily named medically appropriate reasons for seeking ED treatment, such as severe pain, broken bones, seizures, and conditions (stroke, gunshot wounds, and the like) that respondents did not think they could treat—and indeed should not treat—at home. However, just as readily they named concerns such as colds, rashes, small cuts, gynecological issues, and foot pain that were more appropriately treated outside of the ED. The interviews were daunting because, despite their understanding, respondents highlighted several important reasons they continued to use ED for non-emergent reasons, providing some helpful but challenging direction as the hospital taskforce attempted to reduce non-emergent ED usage by Medicaid patients.

Foremost among these factors was a lack of awareness of existing alternatives in the community. This became poignantly evident during a meeting to draft the interview questions when one faith community leader involved in the project expressed surprise to learn that there actually was an immediate care clinic on the campus of the hospital, located near one of the community's hot zones. Although she worked closely with her church's outreach efforts to persons receiving Medicaid, she had (mis) understood the nearest immediate care clinic to be miles away on the more affluent east side of the community. Moreover, when shown to the immediate care clinic, located just a few hundred yards from the ED, she was stunned to discover that the clinic shared office space with her own primary care physician's practice. As survey responses bore out this anecdote, the taskforce realized that raising awareness of alternatives to the ED needed to be an initial priority. Thus, by replacing a poorly visible typewritten sheet of paper that had been taped to the door of the primary care clinic, the hospital harvested some proverbial low-hanging fruit by investing in a larger, more prominent electronic sign announcing the immediate care clinic's hours on the outside of the building, as well as more conspicuous directional signs inside the medical center. Additionally, in recognition that many Medicaid patients lacked the technological resources to be attracted by digital marketing efforts, the hospital printed fliers listing addresses, hours, and directions (including bus routes) for existing immediate care clinics. These fliers were distributed to local churches, particularly those with outreach ministries such as food pantries.

A second, albeit more complex, theme that emerged from the interviews was that a lack of access to alternatives to the ED was a significant barrier for many Medicaid patients in the community. One factor affecting access was transportation— a day-to-day challenge for those who cannot afford reliable vehicles. The issue took on urgency for the taskforce when the local transit authority (under pressure itself to operate as cost-effectively as possible) began considering route changes. In this instance, the hospital successfully argued against the move as proposed and was committed to the construction of a shelter near the hospital. The bus stop issue, however, was a relatively quicker and simple problem to address compared to the deeper problem of finding medical homes for Medicaid patients who were using the ED for primary care because of a limited number of physicians in the community who accepted Medicaid. Although some respondents noted personal familiarity with the ED physicians and trust in the quality of service and care at the ED as reasons for seeking care there, neither EDs nor immediate care clinics can address the continuity of care issue due to the one-off, episodic nature of their context. And while Medicaid patients now are assigned primary care physicians automatically, the hospital's care management team has seen a continued need to work with patients to arrange for transportation to primary care offices or even help them find a new primary care physician in some instances.

Similarly, as hard as the hospital worked to address the issue of non-emergent ED usage by Medicaid patients, one of the big takeaways from the work of the taskforce is that there may be no single solution to the problem, nor can any single discipline or institution resolve the problem on its own. One step that the hospital took to broaden the conversation, for example, was to share the outcomes of the study on ED utilization by Medicaid patients with the Delegate Church Association. As a result, the faith communities decided to focus their thrice-annual meetings and intervening service work on the priorities identified by the federally mandated Community Health Needs Assessment and an implementation plan that is a rare coordinated effort of both local hospitals, a federally qualified health center, and the county health department. For two cycles, the community has made a concerted effort to address the issue of access to care, with one program alone accounting for more than $2 million in annual savings attributable to preventing unnecessary ED visits by Medicaid and working poor patients.

Certainly, other problems remain daunting for Medicaid beneficiaries, including a lack of ready access to willing providers and the complications this presents for coordinated care.

However, by instituting some relatively low-tech steps discussed here, my colleagues were able to nudge what can be a complicated but enormously beneficial public aid program and those who use it into a healthier direction.

The Rev. Mollie Ward is board certified by the Association of Professional Chaplains and is a Certified Educator with the Association for Clinical Pastoral Education. An Episcopal priest with nearly two decades of experience in health care ministry, she holds a master of divinity degree from Seabury-Western Theological Seminary. She is Director of Mission & Spiritual Care, Carle-BroMenn Medical Center, Normal, Illinois.

Medicaid Expansion: Nationalized Politics Meets Intergovernmental Reform
Philip Rocco, PhD

If the Affordable Care Act (ACA) is remembered as an inflection point in the expansion of access to health insurance in the United States, much of the credit should be assigned to the law's expansion of Medicaid coverage. Of the 21 million people who gained insurance coverage within 10 years of the law's passage, more than half received it because of Medicaid expansion. Under the ACA, states could receive unprecedentedly generous federal matching funds to finance the expansion of coverage to Americans whose incomes are below 138 percent of the Federal Poverty Level. The effects of the expansion on health outcomes have been profound. Between 2014 and 2017, one study estimated that states expanding Medicaid cumulatively saved 19,200 lives. Beyond mortality, Medicaid improved utilization of primary care and screenings for low-income adults and treatments for chronic conditions such as cancer and diabetes. New Medicaid enrollees were significantly less likely than their peers in non-expansion states to report skipping medications due to cost. Hospitals in expansion states also saw a dramatic decrease in uncompensated care.

Yet although Medicaid expansion is arguably the ACA's greatest policy success, its implementation also reveals some of the limitations of traditional theories of intergovernmental relations. These theories emphasize that intergovernmental collaboration depends largely on the selection of appropriate fiscal and administrative tools. Evidence from the Medicaid expansion, by contrast, suggests that states' choices about collaboration are embedded within wider political ecologies. Policy choices have been driven not merely by fiscal incentives or administrative negotiations, but by changes in state politics *as a field of institutional power*. States are no longer merely sites of particularized or parochial struggle. Nor do state officials represent their interests before Congress or the Supreme Court in purely functional or fiscal terms. Rather, states have been swept up in national tides of partisan and ideological mobilization. National associations based on pluralistic or professional principles have given way to networks with explicit ideological aims. These networks, mobilized across multiple arenas of power, work to reshape the structure of state-federal relations and the incentives of elected officials to expand Medicaid. At the same time, in the 10 years since the ACA's passage, partisan sorting in the electorate has helped to synchronize state elections to national political trends—contributing to gains for the law's political opponents. In less competitive states, where Medicaid expansion has been off the table, what has mattered is whether voters can successfully localize the issue, shifting the arena of competition through ballot initiatives. Even in these cases, however, legal challenges and federal waivers make the nationalization of the states as a competitive institutional field visible. The upshot here is that ensuring the effective implementation of national reforms requires attention to political variables that are all too often bracketed from intergovernmental policy analysis.

While the ACA represents a modest version of health reform, it passed along strict partisan lines in one of the most ideologically polarized moments in American history.

Few who drafted the law could have foreseen the "shellacking" Democrats would receive in the 2010 midterm elections, yet they clearly understood that implementing the law would not be easy. The starkest evidence of this can be found in the structure of the Medicaid expansion's financing provisions. Historically, the federal government has picked up an average of 57 percent of the cost of Medicaid, with state governments financing the remainder through their own revenue collections. Under the ACA, the federal government agreed to pay 100 percent of state Medicaid costs for newly eligible individuals (those with incomes up to 138 percent of the FPL) for the first four years of implementation. After that, the matching rate tapered to 90 percent in 2020, where it will remain into the foreseeable future. The benefits for state officials seemed obvious: millions of new Medicaid beneficiaries financed almost entirely from federal tax collections, a virtually unprecedented economic multiplier effect, and a new source of stability for hospitals with large uncompensated care costs. If these benefits were not enough, the original legislation made the expansion virtually mandatory by threatening to revoke states' existing Medicaid funding if they refused to accept the expansion.

However politically astute, this last provision invited a swift and highly coordinated response from 26 Republican attorneys general, governors, the National Federation of Independent Business (NFIB), and several individuals. Within minutes of the law's signing ceremony, lawsuits were filed in the federal district court challenging both the Medicaid expansion and the ACA's individual coverage mandate. The Court's decision on Medicaid expansion in *NFIB v. Sebelius* (2012) came as a surprise to many legal academics and observers. A 7-2 majority—which included liberal Justices Stephen Breyer and Elena Kagan—held that the requirement that states participate in Medicaid expansion or risk losing federal funding was a constitutionally impermissible "gun to the head," to quote Chief Justice Roberts' colorful turn of phrase.

The *NFIB* decision had the effect of making the expansion an "opt in" but leaving the ACA's lucrative fiscal and economic incentives in place. Yet, however attractive on paper, these material incentives clashed with the partisan and ideological realities of a more nationalized state politics. During the 2010 midterm elections, conservative backlash at the Obama administration spilled over to the states. The number of states with unified Republican government doubled, enabling coordinated efforts to redistrict state legislatures in Republicans' favor. In the absence of strong electoral competition, the debate over Medicaid expansion was in many states dominated by conservative network organizations such as the American Legislative Exchange Council, which urged Republican governors and state legislators to steadfastly refuse Medicaid dollars. In some cases, as Alex Hertel-Fernandez and colleagues have shown, this pressure ran counter to the demands of political stalwarts in state-level business lobbies and hospital associations.

In the absence of these coordinated national forces, Medicaid expansion might have been a *fait accompli*. Yet Republican governors and legislators now faced a delicate challenge: forgo a federal windfall or risk "guilt by association" with what Republican strategist Frank Luntz had dubbed "Obamacare." In electorally competitive states, Republicans more readily accepted expansion. This was especially true, as Colleen Grogan and Sunggeun Park have shown, in states with larger white populations. While Nevada Governor Brian Sandoval (R) opposed the ACA's individual coverage mandate, for example, he became the first governor in his party to accept Medicaid expansion and to be an intense defender of the expansion when Congress initiated efforts to repeal the law in 2017. The political risk of expansion is stronger for Republicans in less competitive states and states where conservative political networks are better developed. While Alabama Governor Robert Bentley (R) appointed a task force that ultimately recommended Medicaid expansion in 2015, he faced strong legislative opposition, but he was not likely to experience electoral punishment for failure to expand Medicaid. He ultimately abandoned plans to push the proposal forward.

While the interest-group landscape shapes governors' incentives, preexisting institutional legacies structure their opportunities for enacting Medicaid expansion, as Daniel Béland, Philip Rocco, and Alex Waddan have shown. In Wisconsin, Governor Scott Walker (R) drew up an alternative proposal to the full expansion—scaling up eligibility in an existing Medicaid waiver program up to 100 percent of the FPL. This allowed Walker to reject "Obamacare" while claiming that he had "reduce[d] the number of uninsured in [Wisconsin] by 224,580" and added "82,000 people currently living in poverty [to Medicaid]." In Ohio, by contrast, Gov. John Kasich (R) minimized political risk by circumventing opponents in the state legislature. Kasich requested that the state's seven-member Controlling Board, which is charged with overseeing state expenditures, approve the use of federal Medicaid expansion dollars, thereby avoiding a legislative battle.

Policy legacies also helped to reshape the design of the Medicaid expansion across the states. Republican political leaders in states such as Indiana and Arkansas packaged the expansion as part of earlier conservative reforms to the Medicaid program, requesting federal (Section 1115) waivers to impose cost-sharing, benefit restrictions, and work requirements on Medicaid beneficiaries. The outcomes of these proposals, however, depended largely on how they integrated with national governing objectives. With the exception of work requirements, the Obama Administration accepted most of these proposed revisions in exchange for increasing the national rate of insurance coverage. The Trump Administration, by contrast, saw the states as laboratories for experimenting with Medicaid retrenchment. In 2018, the Centers for Medicare and Medicaid Services (CMS) signaled that it would accept waiver applications imposing draconian work requirements not only on the expansion population but also on large slices of the traditional Medicaid population. While more than a dozen states submitted work requirements applications, litigation to enjoin their implementation ensued. In a unanimous opinion, the D.C. Circuit Court of Appeals found that the Trump Administration had—in approving work requirements—neglected Medicaid's core statutory objectives and ignored the effects of the requirements on coverage. In the only state that did implement work requirements, Arkansas, nearly 1 in 4 people subject to the new rules lost coverage over the course of seven months.

As the battle over Section 1115 waivers shows, the nationalization of Medicaid politics has helped to frustrate the course of expansion through the entrenchment of conflict. At the same time, "getting to yes" in states where partisan opposition is strong has also necessitated redirecting the course of the expansion and reinforcing the elements of the program that reduce eligibility. Yet in a number of states, voters have taken another approach to re-localizing the debate over Medicaid expansion: taking it to the ballot box.

Ballot initiatives have emerged as an important mechanism to expand Medicaid in states where governors or state legislatures oppose it. This allows voters to engage in conflict expansion, transforming the decision from an inter-partisan squabble among elected officials into a referendum on a broadly popular benefit. Of course, voters face barriers here too. Only four of the states that have not yet expanded Medicaid give voters the ability to decide this issue at the ballot box. Even where ballot initiatives are allowed, there are procedural hurdles. To qualify for the ballot in the non-expansion state of Wyoming, an initiative must receive a number of signatures equal to 15 percent of votes cast in the previous general election. Second, passage of an initiative requires the support of a majority of voters in the election, rather than just a majority of those voting on the initiative. If an initiative fails to pass, it cannot reappear on the ballot for five years.

More troublingly, as Philip Rocco, Ann Keller, and Andrew Kelly have shown, passage of Medicaid expansion at the ballot box has not been a guarantee of implementation. When

59 percent of Maine voters approved a 2017 Medicaid expansion ballot measure, Governor Paul LePage (R) simply refused to implement the expansion. It took not only lengthy legal battle but also the election of Governor Janet Mills (D) in 2018 for implementation to begin. Other states saw variations on the same obstructive theme. Following Nebraska voters' approval of Medicaid expansion, Governor Pete Ricketts (R) announced that the state would develop an alternative to the plan approved by voters, which would include work requirements and other eligibility restrictions. In Idaho, lawmakers passed an alternative to the Medicaid expansion plan approved by a supermajority of voters. Because the Centers for Medicare and Medicaid Services (CMS) had not yet approved Idaho's legislative alternative, which included both work requirements and a market alternative to Medicaid, Idaho's expansion went into effect as planned in November 2019. Nevertheless, as of March 2020, Idaho's application for a work requirement waiver remained pending before CMS. To be sure, even when governors and legislatures adopted alternatives to voter-approved expansions, Medicaid ballot initiatives did alter the status quo policy. Yet these cases provide a sobering lesson about institutional barriers to voter-led efforts to localize the issue of Medicaid expansion.

The effects of Medicaid expansion on health outcomes are clear. As Benjamin Sommers has illustrated, a state's decision to expand Medicaid translated into one life saved for every 239–316 adults gaining insurance. Numerous studies have documented positive effects of the expansion on access to care, care quality, affordability, and patient outcomes. Yet as of this writing, in the midst of the COVID-19 pandemic, 14 states have not yet expanded Medicaid coverage. More than two million people now fall in the so-called "coverage gap" because they earn too much to qualify for traditional Medicaid but not enough to qualify for the ACA's premium tax credits for the purchase of individual-market coverage. The reasons for this have less to do with the traditional variables of interest in the study of federal-state reforms, such as policy design and the intergovernmental relations of professional administrators. Rather, they are the result of political variables too often bracketed from policy analysis: the organization of political coalitions, the competitiveness of elections, the institutionalization of direct democracy, the strength of voter-led mobilization, the ambitions of national presidential administrations, and so on. The evidence here suggests that—while there are significant economic and health benefits for states' adoption of Medicaid expansion—the nationalization of political conflict has frustrated the traditional logic of intergovernmental policy adoption. The states are less laboratories of democracy than battlefields in a national partisan war—a war in which vulnerable patients are the casualties.

Philip Rocco is an Assistant Professor of Political Science at Marquette University. He specializes in American politics, with a focus on federalism, public policy, and the political economy of policy knowledge. He is the co-author of Obamacare Wars: Federalism, State Politics, and the Affordable Care Act *(University Press of Kansas, 2016) and co-editor of* American Political Development and the Trump Presidency *(University of Pennsylvania Press, 2020). His work has appeared in journals such as* Political Science Quarterly; Journal of Health Politics, Policy, and Law; Health Affairs; *and the* Journal of Public Policy.

Medicare from an Enrollee's Perspective
Ann C.

In the autumn of 2012, I enrolled in traditional Medicare. Instead of feeling old and vulnerable—after all, I was about to turn 65—I felt relieved that I would now be able to use Medicare, a program I had paid into during my working years. My friends and I, who were the same age, were nearly celebratory on reaching this milestone. We couldn't be rejected for coverage. Rather, we would now be become part of a government program that would pay for the majority of our health needs. Medicare, of course, is not free. In my case, the government deducts my costs for Parts B and D and then deposits the remainder in my checking account. This has all worked smoothly from the time I enrolled in 2012.

In addition, I have secondary medical and drug insurance policies. On several occasions, I have changed insurance companies when my insurance advisor found medical or drug policies with more reasonable premiums. With my additional secondary policies and Medicare, I feel confident that my health care payments will be covered for the rest of my life. With health care costs constantly rising, that could be an expensive proposition for the U.S. government. Without this coverage, it would certainly be an expensive proposition for me.

In addition to paying for doctors' office visits and procedures, Medicare pays for a yearly "wellness" visit with my internist. On occasion, he has recommended a lab test not covered by Medicare. I have always followed his recommendations and paid for these tests out of pocket. How Medicare decides which tests are worthy of reimbursement is unknown to me. Each year I have a mammogram, paid for by Medicare, and a flu shot. Medicare has paid for several colonoscopies, which are recommended every 10 years. Fortunately, I have received negative results from these procedures and subsequently felt relieved. However, I presume, these proactive measures have saved lives and mitigated future costs for Medicare.

Having remarked above that I am relatively healthy, I now admit to a weakness. I have worn out my joints. I had a hip replacement, knee replacement, and minor surgery on my right foot, all after going on Medicare. Medicare and my secondary insurance paid for these expensive procedures. In addition, Medicare paid for physical therapy after the hip and knee replacements. Through physical therapy, I was able to heal more quickly and learn about my new prosthetics from knowledgeable therapists. I am grateful for all this care and the bills paid by Medicare and my secondary insurance.

Having reviewed my experience with Medicare, I conclude that my initial relief for going on Medicare was justified. My expenses, deducted from Social Security, have not been overly burdensome. I have sought out the best care I could find, and Medicare has paid for the majority of the costs for necessary procedures and consultations. They have generously paid for preventive services, such as the annual flu shot. So far, Medicare has helped me stay healthy and active.

Ann C. is a Medicare beneficiary and a retired educator. Her experiences with the program services are approximately in line with those of typical enrollees her age. Like some 80 percent of seniors on Medicare, she has a supplemental health insurance policy to cover the gaps left by her government insurance.

The Growing Privatization of Medicare
Andrew Scholnick

American social policy is continuously balancing communal responsibility against individual choice. Health care policy, in particular, is a philosophical tug-of-war regarding the role of government in keeping a person healthy. At the heart of each new idea to ensure Americans have access to affordable health coverage—whether it's Medicare and Medicaid in 1965, catastrophic coverage in 1988, prescription drug coverage in 2003, or the Affordable Care Act in 2010—lies a debate between those who support government action to correct market inefficiencies and those who think it's best to let the marketplace sort itself out. The policy of push and pull continues even when the law is well established and settled. Even now, as debates play out regarding government-run insurance and expanding Medicare to everyone, Medicare itself is becoming increasingly more privatized.

Historical Trends toward Privatization

As originally conceived, Medicare is a health care plan that pays for hospital services (Part A) and physician services and post-acute care (Part B) for people aged 65 or older and younger persons with disabilities. The benefits and covered services are essentially the same across the country, there are no provider networks to worry about, and clinicians get paid roughly the same amount no matter what Medicare patients they see. (There is some variation on payment rates based on regional price differences, which are calculated by the Geographic Practice Cost Index. Also, while traditional Medicare has a standard benefit and baseline of covered services, regional Medicare Administrative Contractors are able to make local coverage determinations for services that are not expressly covered by Medicare.) Furthermore, when Medicare was created, everyone paid the same premiums and faced the same costs. Today, premiums are income related, and there are programs to help low-income individuals with premiums and cost-sharing. The egalitarian nature of Medicare—in which everyone is treated essentially the same—is one of its defining features and engenders widespread support. However, tension arises between the "we" and the "me." While traditional Medicare provides a strong foundation and baseline of coverage, it is not necessarily perfect for every individual. Many people purchase supplemental coverage (also known as Medigap) to help potentially high out-of-pocket costs, need standalone plans for services that are not covered by original Medicare (e.g., dental and vision services), and have to purchase prescription drug coverage. What if one wanted additional covered services or was willing to accept a limited provider network or other restrictions in exchange for lower costs? The standard Medicare plan might be good for the collective "we", but it may not work for each individual "me." The challenge for legislators and policy makers is balancing what the individual wants versus what is good public policy.

Partly in response to this desire for more individualized coverage, officials have let private insurers operate in conjunction with or alongside Medicare. These private insurance plans are paid by Medicare to provide Medicare coverage to Medicare beneficiaries. Over time, more and more privatization has crept into Medicare. Beginning in the 1970s, CMS began allowing private plans to contract with Medicare. In 1982, Medicare started offering capitated payments to private health plans to provide coverage for Part A and Part B. By 1997, these plans were formalized into Medicare Part C, the Medicare+Choice program. In 2003, reimbursement rates were changed, and the program was reformed and renamed Medicare Advantage (MA). Medicare Part D was created the same year, offering prescription drug coverage exclusively through subsidized private insurance plans, not government-administered coverage. MA plans could incorporate Part D drug coverage into their Part C plan offerings. Under Part D, not only was responsibility for covering prescription drugs ceded to private insurers, but also the government was expressly prohibited from using the bargaining power of 60 million beneficiaries to negotiate for lower drug prices, under what is known as the noninterference clause of the Medicare Modernization Act. Unlike in Part A and Part B where Medicare has more authority to set prices for services and drugs, Part D leaves prices and costs up to the market. Over time, the divergent policies of MA from original Medicare led to MA plans being overpaid by about 13 percent relative to the cost of original Medicare. The Affordable Care Act of 2010 changed the reimbursement structure to make payments to MA plans more in line with the cost of original Medicare, while solidifying MA's place in our health care system. Today, just over one-third of all Medicare beneficiaries are enrolled in a Medicare Advantage plan.

Some legislators and policy makers believe Medicare's reliance on private plans should be expanded even further. In this view, private health plans are not a means to an end (i.e., affordable health coverage), but the end itself. Adherents of this view argue that because MA is increasingly popular, all Medicare beneficiaries should be in it. Ideologically, they believe that private insurers can better administer coverage than the government and that it will be cheaper for taxpayers. Thus, there have been repeated attempts to change Medicare into a "premium-support" or "defined contribution" program, which provides vouchers to beneficiaries to purchase a private plan.

This would eliminate the guaranteed benefit currently enjoyed by Medicare beneficiaries.

It is hard to ignore the role of insurance companies in swaying public policy. Health insurance is big business, and companies see a large untapped market among Medicare beneficiaries. Their efforts have swayed politicians and the public discourse. While attempts to fully privatize Medicare have failed in the face of public backlash, the Medicare program is nevertheless becoming increasingly market-oriented. Deference and preference are often given to Medicare Advantage over traditional Medicare, whether an individual is working through an agent or broker or reviewing plans themselves on the Medicare. gov plan finder. Most notably, Medicare Advantage plans are being allowed to offer benefits that traditional Medicare is not allowed to offer.

Recent Developments toward Privatization

Medicare Advantage plans have been allowed to offer supplemental benefits, such as hearing, dental, and vision coverage, for many years. Until recently, these benefits had to be primarily health related, though. Consumers may also be charged an additional amount for that coverage, and the same extra benefits had to be available to everyone enrolled in that plan. More recently, as a result of the Bipartisan Budget Act of 2018, MA plans can now offer a wider array of supplemental services. Moreover, plans can tailor benefits to enrollees and offer special non-health-related benefits for people with chronic conditions. (Considerable research into supplemental benefit offerings has been done by Jane Sung and Claire Noel-Miller of AARP's Public Policy Institute. See www.aarp.org for further information.)

As with any change to public policy, there are positive and negative tradeoffs. On the one hand, Medicare beneficiaries could have much greater access to needed services, such as meals, transportation, or home improvements to prevent falls. The new rules removed barriers and restrictions, thereby letting MA plans make coverage available to more people. MA plans can also choose to offer support for family caregivers, such as education and respite. The hope and expectation is that these additional services will lead to more comprehensive and better managed care.

On the other hand, offering supplemental benefits is optional for MA plans. Not all beneficiaries will have the opportunity to buy plans in their area. Plus, those who do have a choice of plans in their area may be overwhelmed and confused by the variation in plan offerings. There is growing evidence that, on the whole, seniors are not particularly active shoppers when it comes to selecting Medicare coverage. For example, we know that Medicare beneficiaries generally do not change their plans during open enrollment each year, so it is unlikely that most people will take advantage of the opportunity to find new coverage with benefits that suit their particular needs. Even if Medicare beneficiaries choose the coverage, we do not know how meaningful these new benefits will be for consumers. Plans could promote supplemental benefits to attract customers, but offer very little value. Moreover, under the new rules, not everyone in the plan may be eligible for the benefits because the plans no longer have to offer uniform coverage to all plan participants. If policy makers believe these supplemental benefits are effective at improving care or lowering overall cost, then they should be covered by Medicare across the board.

Allowing MA to offer supplemental benefits makes those plans more attractive to consumers compared to traditional Medicare. Two-thirds of Medicare beneficiaries, roughly 40 million people, have traditional Medicare, and they are not offered these benefits. The comparative market advantage could accelerate the migration of individuals from traditional Medicare to Medicare Advantage plans, leaving behind people who are unable to change. The challenge for policy makers and legislators is to ensure all beneficiaries have robust, high-quality coverage, whether it's through traditional Medicare or private Medicare Advantage plans.

Andrew Scholnick is a health policy professional focused on Medicare, currently representing AARP before Congress and the Administration. He has over 15 years of experience advocating on behalf of health care organizations, such as the American Cancer Society, the Cancer Action Network, and the American Academy of Otolaryngology–Head and Neck Surgery. His opinion and expertise have been quoted by numerous national and local media outlets, including the Washington Post, USA Today, *and* CNBC.com.

The American Health Care State
Robert Y. Shapiro, PhD

Despite all the noisy opposition voiced by Republican opponents of the Affordable Care Act over the past decade, and particularly by President Trump since his inauguration, these opponents have probably done more to solidify public support for government efforts in health care than have traditional progressive backers of government health insurance in recent years. There is a case to be made that the more Obamacare foes try to undermine the 2010 law, the more Americans tune in to finally appreciate the many things government does for them and to resist efforts to backtrack on the progress made, particularly in reducing the percentage of people living without health insurance. Beyond revealing this irony, recent fights over health care have also shone a light on the ability of the public to learn at least some of what it needs to know about its own health care.

Looking back to earlier years, the original enactment and implementation of the Social Security, Medicare, and Medicaid entitlement programs enabled Democratic presidential administrations to establish and provide a firm political grounding for the American *welfare state*, a broad but inconsistent network of programs designed to help and protect the most vulnerable. As important subsidiaries of this safety net, the Medicare and Medicaid programs are the main components of the American *health care state*. Over time, Americans have come to take these programs for granted and enjoy the many ways Medicare and Medicaid provide security in the face of often unexpected adversity. As beneficial as they are, Medicare and Medicaid still leave a lot of coverage gaps. The Affordable Care Act, passed in March 2010, was President Barack Obama's and congressional Democrats' attempt to expand the health care state, filling some of these gaps. The passage was remarkable, given the strong opposition from Republican politicians and deep misgivings, often downright opposition, of many citizens. These misgivings reflected the public's longstanding skepticism of—not simply ambivalence toward— nationalized health care in the United States. Of course, this skepticism has existed alongside the public's strong support for, not merely a practical dependence on, Medicare for the elderly and disabled, as well as Medicaid for those living in or near poverty.

Just as the American welfare state anchored by the three entitlement programs became fully established when they were, sometimes grudgingly, accepted by subsequent Republican administrations, the health care state has, ironically, been strengthened during President Donald Trump's administration. This has occurred through a political learning process for citizens and policy makers alike that eluded the Obama Administration during its time. The law's architects had fully expected that the public would soon support the reforms provided by the ACA when it saw the improvements that this change in national health care policy provided. Prominently, they believed states would readily adopt the Medicaid expansion that came with a promise of nearly complete federal funding. It turns out they were wrong. That learning did not occur for various reasons, but particularly because the benefits of the ACA did not immediately become visible during a period of a national economic downturn. Public opinion toward the ACA was no more than mixed and declining when it was passed, and it remained an election issue in 2016 when Donald Trump and the other Republican presidential candidates called Obamacare a disaster and promised to *end Obamacare* immediately after they were elected.

It turns out they were wrong too. After Trump's election, the learning process entered a new phase. For one, while Trump wanted to end Obamacare, he promised not to touch any of the major entitlement programs. Second, in following up on his promise to dismantle Obamacare, he kept health care a highly visible national issue and increased the public's attention to it through an almost endless stream of criticism that, for the most part, lacked content about what an alternative set of policies would be. Trump didn't do his policy homework, and apparently, he believed large swaths of the general public wouldn't do theirs either and that they would not think through the downsides of repealing generous insurance subsidies and consumer protections such as those relating to preexisting medical conditions. The negative attention was crucial in that normally the public has not been substantially attuned to all the ways in which government policies make individuals' lives better—owing both to its longstanding skepticism toward government and to its unawareness of all that government does. As political scientist Suzanne Mettler explains in her book, *The Submerged State*, a wide range of social benefits routinely help millions of Americans, but many of them lie virtually invisible and do not get swept up in day-to-day political discourse. A chief consequence is that the government does not get credit for tax deductions that provide subsidies for home owners, student loan guarantees, and retirement savings that constitute income support—effectively "welfare"—for the middle class and the rich, not just those with lower incomes.

This lack of awareness, however, can change through sustained attention, even if the discourse is somewhat chaotic, and many of the messages are crafted to reframe the debate or even manipulate popular understandings of the facts. One source of the unawareness surrounding health care is tied up with skepticism toward government. These distortions arise from partisan conflict in which, for example, Republicans and others opposing the Democrats lose sight of which party supports which benefits. For example, in the heat of opposition against the Obama administration spurred on by the Tea Party movement, there came to be in many quarters an incoherent visceral opposition to all things having to do with the administration, including the ACA, coupled with a gratitude for the government assistance. While the ignorance behind the insistence that "government must keep its hands off my Medicare" is certainly startling, it also reveals a deeper misunderstanding that substantial public learning can only turn around slowly in the face of hyper-partisan discourse. Hence, in the case of the expansion of Medicaid that is part of the ACA, many Kentuckians living in a Republican state that expanded Medicaid eligibility to reach a quarter of its residents can manage to simultaneously complain about Obamacare while also enjoying their newfound Medicaid coverage.

This largely partisan opposition to Obamacare started to change when Trump and the Republican-held Congress tried to terminate the ACA in 2017. The prospect of rolling back the health care state quickly raised the awareness and visibility of what benefits many individuals in need would lose if they lost the medical insurance that they had through Obamacare—whether through the expansion of Medicaid or the insurance exchanges that were subsidized through reduced taxes or refunds. These subsidies were more "submerged" than the new Medicaid insurance people obtained, but a lot of the public evidently became aware of these benefits, especially those who needed this new insurance because of their own or family members' urgent or chronic health problems. As a result of this learning, the additional public support for the ACA that eluded Obama and the Democrats finally emerged, and it pressured enough members of Congress to thwart the repeal of the ACA. The most that Trump and the Republicans could do was to end the ACA's individual insurance mandate (enforced by a tax penalty) that everyone obtain health insurance and later the tax on medical devices and the tax on high-end "Cadillac" insurance plans. These were in parts of the ACA that a majority of the public opposed, so what was left in the ACA were all or nearly all the policies and requirements that were widely supported by Democrats and Republicans alike among the public.

This public learning and the Republican failure thus far to end Obamacare has further entrenched support for the health care state with the heightened salience of this issue. While this has varied over time, a large and more stable majority of Americans believe it is the government's responsibility to do what it can to make sure people have health insurance. Crucially, this has become the new *starting point* for debate over further policy reforms. This is Exhibit A in making the case that public learning can happen, even if catalyzed by years of partisan criticism.

Coming up to the present, Democrats have turned the question of government-enabled health insurance—whether public or private—into a key campaign issue for the 2020 presidential election. The conversation over Medicare for All, or a public insurance option, or something else has a new starting point given the evolution of the American health care state. This new starting point may not be enough to overcome continued public reluctance about universal public insurance in lieu of that provided by employers or private plans, but it certainly makes arguments about rolling back the Medicaid expansion seem like things of the past. A majority of the public support the government for expanding the availability of Medicare and Medicaid, which further shows its deep support for expanding the American health care state.

While Democrats see the expansion of the health care state in the offing, congressional Republicans are not done trying to prevent this and to move in the opposite direction. The Republicans' efforts have focused on federal court cases that could result in a ruling that the 2017 elimination of the individual insurance mandate renders the rest of the ACA invalid. If such a ruling were to win support from the Supreme Court, this would collide with solid public support for what the ACA has provided in expanding the availability and the quality of health insurance, especially for people with preexisting conditions, and it would exert pressure to continue these benefits in some way.

Despite the solidification of the health care state, headwinds persist. While there has been no serious move to retrench the Medicare program, occasional talk of vouchers still comes from some advocates on the Right. However, the actually enacted policy changes passed in 2018 allow Medicare Advantage plans to offer an *enhanced* range of services, which will almost certainly boost public support even further for this broadened component of the health care state. On Medicaid, the Trump Administration has encouraged state-level work requirements for some Medicaid recipients and has talked of turning Medicaid into a block grant program allowing states to deviate from the current required features of the federal program. Even if the movement to turn Medicaid into a block grant were to begin to gain traction, this would almost certainly lead to a debate that would provide the opportunity for Americans to affirm once again their evolving belief in a health care state.

Robert Y. Shapiro is the Wallace S. Sayre Professor of Government in the Department of Political Science and Professor of International and Public Affairs at Columbia University. He specializes in American politics, with a focus on public opinion, policy making, political leadership, the mass media, and research methodology. His books that include analyses of public opinion and health care policy are The Rational Public *(with Benjamin Page) and* Politicians Don't Pander *(with Lawrence Jacobs).*

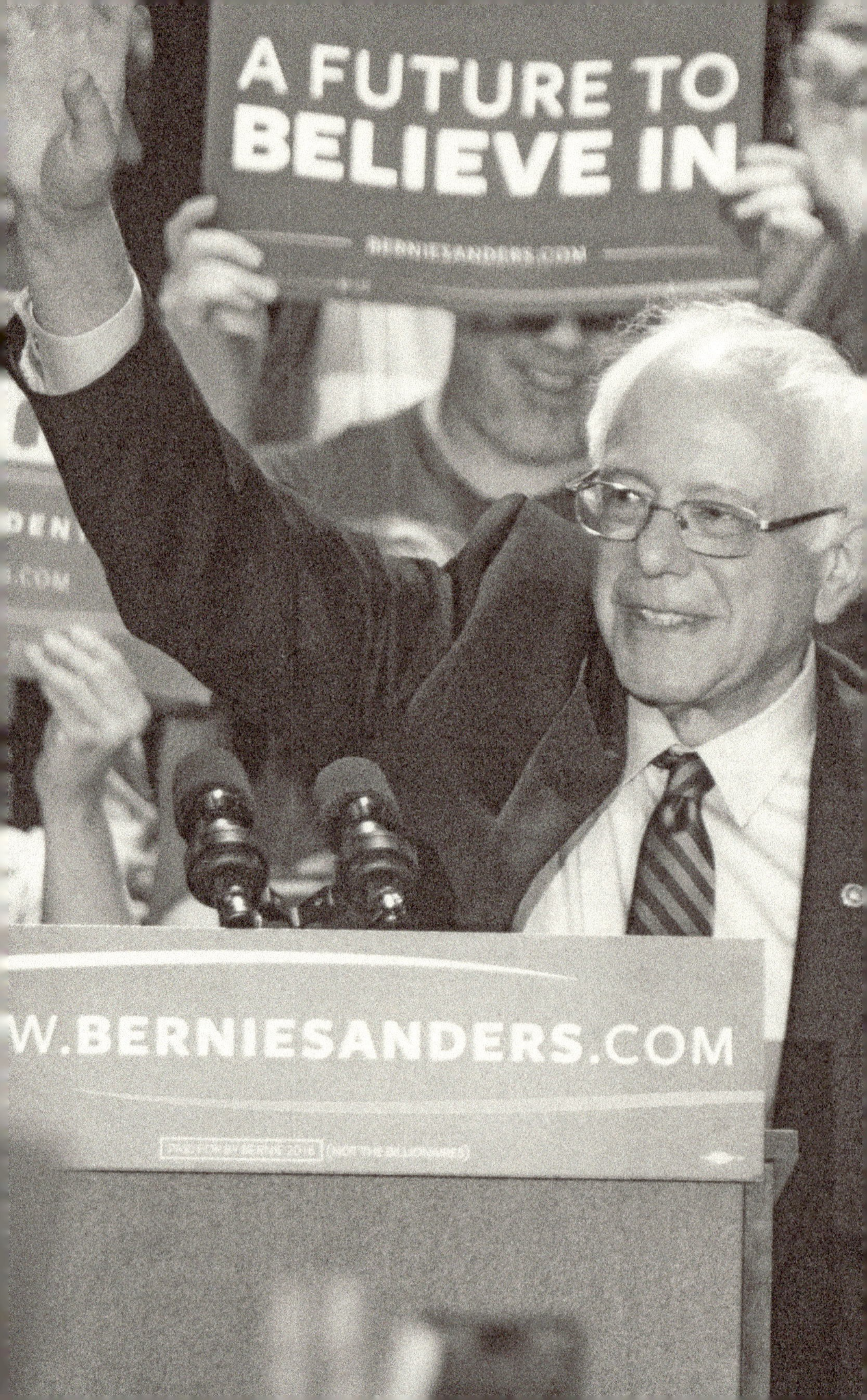
A FUTURE TO
BELIEVE IN
BERNIESANDERS.COM
W.BERNIESANDERS.COM

4 Profiles of People and Organizations

Introduction

This chapter profiles individuals and organizations that advocate on Medicare and Medicaid. These groups range from large health insurance companies to nonprofit research organizations, to industry and physician groups, to small but exuberant policy shops, to politicians and other government officials. The American Medical Association (AMA), founded in 1847, is the oldest organization profiled here. In contrast, the Partnership for America's Health Care Future was formed in 2018. Several of these groups annually spend tens of millions of dollars on their efforts, while others mainly focus on street-level activism by their followers around the country. Some of these groups are umbrella organizations made up of other entities for the purpose of applying pressure on Medicare or Medicaid policy. Several of them, such as the U.S. Chamber of Commerce and the American Hospital Association (AHA), routinely collaborate with others. Others function more independently. The Centers for Medicare and Medicaid Services (CMS) is the federal agency responsible for administering these two programs. The organizations appear alphabetically below. Source material was taken from the organizations' websites and published academic

U.S. Senator Bernie Sanders campaigns for president. Though unsuccessful at securing the Democratic nomination, Sanders has convinced many Americans to support Medicare for All. (Danny Raustadt/Dreamstime.com)

and media reports. Figures on political contributions come from the nonpartisan Center for Responsive Politics. Select sources appear at the end of this chapter.

The American Hospital Association

The AHA, the nation's largest hospital lobbying group, represents nearly 5,000 hospitals and other health care organizations on both the for-profit and not-for-profit sides of the industry. Founded in 1899 in Cleveland, Ohio, the Association acted during its early years essentially as a private club for hospital superintendents. However, it evolved to address a wider range of concerns, and for decades, it has engaged in both political advocacy and the development and promotion of professional best practices. The Association now has offices in Chicago and Washington, D.C. Reflecting its strong focus on political advocacy, the AHA has convened its annual meetings in the nation's capital since 1970 as a way of connecting its membership with policy makers on a regular basis. This work has involved legislative lobbying, executive branch liaison, as well as litigation and submission of amicus briefs before the federal courts, such as it did in the important 2015 case of *King v. Burwell*. In this instance, the Supreme Court agreed that the Affordable Care Act (ACA) requires federal subsidies to individuals who purchase insurance on either state or federal exchanges. This ruling aligned with the AHA's preference.

The AHA's positions over the past several decades arguably have been less ideologically strident than those of many other groups representing sectors of organized medicine. In the early 1960s, it supported the ideas that would become Medicare and Medicaid before the AMA did, and in recent years, it has adopted a pragmatic posture in its political advocacy, defending existing federal programs instead of waging the symbolic and ideological battles that have consumed many other lobbying organizations. A unifying theme in its public messaging since the passage of the ACA has focused on the importance of maximizing health insurance coverage for those individuals who have traditionally lacked it. Given that hospitals face the main brunt of uncompensated care resulting from uninsured and under-insured persons, this focus speaks directly to AHA members' financial health. Attributable to Medicare and Medicaid alone, this burden amounted to just over $76 billion in 2017, according to the Association's analysis (American Hospital Association 2019).

While some uncompensated care arises on the private insurance side of hospital financing, Medicare and Medicaid are the main drivers of this problem. Based on an analysis of 2017 data, the AHA found that, on average, hospitals received only 87 cents for each dollar they spent on care from both of these programs. As explained in Chapter 2, throughout its history Medicare has reimbursed providers at levels that usually do not quite allow them to break even financially on these patients. For its part, Medicaid provides even less, though Disproportionate Share Hospital payments bring the gross Medicaid underpayment rate into approximate parity with the closer-to-adequate Medicare underpayment rate. Naturally, the fact that both programs pay less than the cost of service provision leads the AHA routinely to advocate for maintaining and expanding Medicare payment levels, which the ACA slated for gradual reduction through the 2010s (American Hospital Association 2019). This will continue to be a conflict for the foreseeable future.

Strongly in support of the ACA's Medicaid expansion, the leadership of the AHA has called for all states to expand their Medicaid programs in the interest of maximizing health insurance coverage. In its 2018 Advocacy Agenda document, it advanced the idea of state-level insurance mandates for individuals, the federal version of which was the most controversial element of the ACA. It has also urged the Department of Health and Human Services to guarantee that newly expanding states complete federal funding for their expansion population for three full years, an offer that went off the table for states that declined to expand Medicaid eligibility in 2014. Federal funding still covers 90 percent of the expansion population costs under the ACA. The Association clearly wants to minimize the number of uninsured people who show up on their members' doorsteps, regardless of state lawmakers' partisan objections to the ACA.

At a time when scores of hospitals have closed, largely due to financial crises, the AHA's support for government insurance programs speaks directly to these concerns. The issues go beyond simply asking for larger Medicare payments under its various schedules, such as the Hospital Inpatient Prospective Payment System (under Part A) and the Hospital Outpatient Prospective Payment System (under Part B). The Association has also challenged Medicare innovations designed to foster more efficient service delivery. For instance, under the ACA, hospitals and their affiliated groups of providers were invited to form Accountable Care Organizations. When these groups were able to deliver quality care to their geographic client populations and to do so efficiently, they shared in the savings, often receiving millions of dollars per year in special payments. However, the challenges involved in these initiatives led the AHA to critique the project, saying that it involved too much risk for hospitals and not enough financial reward.

As a second example of challenging a Medicare policy that was designed to instill regularity and transparency into billing practices, the AHA sued the CMS in 2014 over the Two Midnight Rule, which stipulates that, with a few exceptions, any hospital stay that lasts less than two midnights must be billed on an outpatient (meaning lower-paying) basis. The AHA took the position that this rule is arbitrary and that CMS violated the federal Administrative Procedures Act by not providing hospitals sufficient time to respond to the proposed rule. Far from complaining about "Washington takeovers" of health care, such as those that were a staple of conservative politicians and their allies during the creation of the ACA and the law's early years, the AHA has been very willing to play the game of government insurance, and it works doggedly to maximize those payments to its member hospitals and clinics.

Beyond Medicare and Medicaid, the AHA wants to see the online Marketplace and its federally funded subsidies expand beyond the current ceiling of 400 percent of the federal poverty level. Elevating that eligibility threshold would provide for potentially generous tax credits for solidly middle-class families, and while this would likely generate some political controversy, it would essentially mimic the tax break that employers and their workers receive under the preferential tax treatment of employer-provided health insurance. This idea, though it is not fully elaborated in the AHA's recent advocacy documents, represents something of a middle way between broadening Medicaid even further and the public insurance option touted by a number of prominent Democrats and their progressive supporters.

Because the AHA knows it cannot count on Medicare and Medicaid payments alone to balance its members' budgets, it also defends a robust employer-based insurance subscribership. The Association's press releases not only highlight the principle of consumer choice but also prominently remind readers of the financial consequences of low-reimbursement government insurance. This, of course, also speaks to the Association's opposition to Medicare for All proposals. Rick Pollack, the Association's CEO, picked up on the language of the Partnership for America's Health Care Future (also profiled in this chapter), a consortium to which the AHA belongs, as he referred to Medicare for All as an unhelpful instance of one-size-fits-all insurance (Kacik 2017). Pollack pointed out how the "government can be an unreliable business partner" and that the goal should be to bolster stable insurance arrangements that he believes characterize employer-provided coverage better than do public programs (Pollack 2019). In line with this position, Pollack offered his support for the ACA's employer mandate, an element of the 2010 law that has proved to be controversial.

In addition to these educational efforts aimed at a broad audience, the AHA also spends many millions of dollars each year on lobbying federal elected officials and other policy makers in order to drive home these points. According to the Center for Responsive Politics, in 2018 alone the AHA spent nearly $24 million on such efforts. The Association does less in the way of direct candidate funding, spending only $2.1 million in 2018. Those contributions benefitted a wide range of federal candidates and included both Democrats and Republicans.

American Medical Association

The AMA is the nation's largest association of physicians. Its mission is to promote the practice of medicine and public health in the United States. Founded in 1847 at a time when medicine was much less formalized than it is today, the AMA spent most of the first half century of its existence struggling against what its leadership considered to be irregular practitioners: homeopaths, chiropractors, osteopaths, primitive psychotherapists, and religious healers, among others, all of whom were, in the AMA's view, quacks and snake oil salesmen. As medical education and practices modernized throughout the early 20th century, the AMA played important roles in formalizing graduate education, licensure, professional norms, and best practices and, importantly, resisting what it saw as government interference in medicine. From the 1930s through at least the 1960s—depending on whom one speaks with—the AMA opposed government-sponsored health insurance, particularly the Social Security-based proposals that percolated among liberal Democrats during the Franklin Roosevelt through John Kennedy administrations. Following the enactment of Medicare and Medicaid in 1965, the leadership of the AMA threatened to boycott the programs, though this resistance gave way over the next few years, as most physicians came to accept the programs as payment for services.

In addition to its political advocacy, the AMA publishes the *Journal of the American Medical Association* (*JAMA*), a prominent venue for research and commentary on medicine. It also publishes the *Physician Specialty Codes*, which identifies physician specialties, and it maintains the *AMA Code of Medical Ethics*. To enable its political involvements, the association supports the American Medical Political Action Committee. Over time, the AMA has become more inclusive. In contrast to how it resisted women in the practice of medicine throughout the latter half of the 19th century, since 2018 it has had three consecutive female presidents.

An important development since the early 1990s has been the AMA's significant warming toward government involvement in health care financing. Whereas it opposed the Clinton plan because it feared greater government involvement in insurance markets would inevitably lead to greater government control over health care delivery, the AMA's leadership did not actively oppose the passage of the ACA. Further, when in 2018 the Partnership for America's Health Care Future formed to oppose Medicare for All proposals, the AMA initially joined but then reversed itself and parted ways from this oppositional group in 2019.

The year 2019 marked a time of transition for the AMA's leadership. In March of that year, the AMA stated that it "is opposed to Medicare for All based on a mountain of evidence about the cost, counterproductive disruption and degradation of choice, quality and innovation that Americans deserve and want" (Japsen 2019a). However, like some other physician associations such as the American College of Physicians and the American Academy of Family Physicians, the AMA supports the idea of broadening public insurance, perhaps through some form of Medicare buy-in or a public insurance option, while maintaining its opposition to a wholesale dismantling of the private insurance industry. Clearly, these provider groups realize the importance of a mix of patients and the payments they bring as an important way to balance their finances.

As the months passed and the AMA endured protests by the group Physicians for a National Heath Program (also profiled here), and reminders from within that many, perhaps most, of its physician members had come to support some type of single-payer system, the AMA rather visibly pulled out of the Partnership for America's Health Care Future, claiming that it instead wanted to focus on practical solutions instead of political conflicts. As diplomatic as this press release language may have been, even more telling of its growing acceptance of government-supported insurance were several articles appearing in *JAMA* during 2018 and 2019 supporting the idea of a single-payer health care system (Fuchs 2018). Clearly, the AMA does not want to share in the political combat that the Partnership for America's Health Care Future is likely to experience over the coming few election cycles.

In support of a mix of types of payment systems, the AMA has advocated for broader subsidies for Americans who purchase their health insurance through the online Marketplace. The doctors' association sees this as a way to provide ample insurance coverage—meaning fewer nonpaying patients—as well as a way to preserve the extensive consumer choice that private insurance provides (in contrast to the narrow networks often associated with Medicaid, for instance). Hoping to see more moderate-income people able to take advantage of tax credits when purchasing insurance, the AMA supports not only an expansion of the upper-income threshold for tax credit eligibility (currently 400% of the federal poverty level) but also to make the credits themselves more generous. In direct opposition to the unpopularity of the individual mandate that was the most controversial element of the ACA (until it was made inoperative effective January of 2019), the AMA supports individual mandates at the state level (American Medical Association 2019). The common theme here is that the AMA wants to maximize insurance coverage, preferably through government subsidies in conjunction with private markets, though it has demonstrated a willingness to support a greater role for government-provided insurance as well.

Illustrating this latter point, the AMA has defended the Medicaid program in general and the ACA's expansion of it in particular. In 2017, the AMA's House of Delegates, its long-standing policy making body, sent Congress a strong message about the importance of preserving the open-ended entitlement basis for Medicaid funding. In response to Republican proposals in Congress during that year to convert Medicaid's funding to a block grant, with fixed annual payments to states, the AMA's leadership opposed this. The specific proposal in question, The American Health Care Act, which passed the House of Representatives in May 2017, would have shifted Medicaid's funding to a block grant within two years. The AMA's House of Delegates doubled down on this issue, adding its voice to the association's earlier report, issued by the AMA's Council on Medical Service, opposing Medicaid block grants.

One other sign that the AMA strongly supports existing government insurance programs was that the association threw its support behind an effort to eliminate the federal Independent Payment Advisory Board, which was created under the ACA as a mechanism to reduce Medicare reimbursements as a way of saving taxpayer money, though at the expense of medical providers. The IPAB proved to be controversial because it would have had the power to cut Medicare payments without those decisions being enacted by a congressional vote. The AMA likened the IPAB to Medicare's sustainable growth rate formula, which was another effort during the 2000s and 20-teens systematically to reduce Medicare's overall expenditure trajectory. The AMA and its supporters on this issue were successful, as the IPAB was eliminated by the Bipartisan Budget Act of 2018.

It is notable that this physician association, whose members are well aware of the inadequacy of Medicaid payments, would so strongly oppose the diminution of a program that it outright opposed years ago. Seeing Medicaid as one part of a complex mix of patients, and given that low payments are better than no payments from some of their patients, the AMA has gradually shifted from being an oppositional force to a reluctant partner, to now playing the role of an adamant supporter of Medicaid.

Strikingly absent from the AMA's recent messaging is the once sweeping opposition to government involvement in financing that for decades its leadership tied to notions of "socialized medicine." Instead, the AMA now recognizes that its members can practice medicine with a robust degree of professional autonomy alongside this government program.

Taking positions on Medicaid and Medicare is one of the many pursuits of the AMA. In 2019, the AMA lobbied on dozens of different issues related to Medicare, Medicaid, and other concerns. Over the past two decades, the AMA typically has spent between $15 and $20 million annually on lobbying, marking it as a major player in Washington, D.C. Its state-level associated groups fulfil similar roles in state capitals (Center for Responsive Politics 2019).

Americans for Prosperity

Founded by the libertarian billionaires Charles and David Koch, owners of Koch Industries and sons of Fred Koch, a founding member of the stridently antigovernment John Birch Society, Americans for Prosperity (AfP) is widely recognized as one of the most influential conservative political organizations in the United States. Formally a not-for-profit group organized under section 501(c)(4) of the Internal Revenue Code, it is not required to reveal its donors, which makes it impossible to say exactly how large its budget is. However, campaign spending reports routinely place these expenditures in the tens of millions of dollars per year (Hertel-Fernandez et al. 2018). AfP, based in Arlington, Virginia, was formed in 2004 when the free-market advocacy group called Citizens for a Sound Economy broke up due to internal philosophical disagreements. The longtime Republican strategist Tim Phillips has served as AfP's president since 2006. As of 2020, AfP has affiliates with paid staff in 36 states. David Koch died in August 2019, but all indications are that his surviving brother will continue supporting the organization at a high level. While this group is one among several organizations sponsored by the Kochs, it is the main platform for their advocacy work.

Americans for Prosperity works on a variety of political issues but is especially well known for waging political warfare against labor unions and the ACA, particularly the Medicaid expansion. Since 2009, AfP has adopted the strategy of mobilizing protests at state capitals and in legislators' town hall meetings, door-knocking and phone banking, and radio, TV, and social media campaigns, among other efforts to sway public opinion. It tends to take oppositional stances on government involvement in health care more often than it advocates for specific legislative proposals. Its spending during the 2018 election cycle illustrates this pattern. During that period, AfP spent over $11 million to defeat Democrats and only $4.2 million to support Republicans (Center for Responsive Politics data). As committed libertarians, the Koch brothers have not always seen eye to eye with Republican office holders, though they have certainly preferred them over Democrats.

Since the beginning, AfP has taken a state-by-state organizational strategy. This has allowed them to build what can look like grassroots pressure on members of Congress as well as state legislators. In several instances, Americans for Prosperity injected large amounts of money into nascent groups with sympathetic political interests. The ramping up of the Tea Party movement during 2008 and 2009 is the most prominent example. While this has earned AfP the reputation among some observers as a manufacturer of astroturf politicking, it has been undeniably successful at both the national and state levels. Americans for Prosperity has sponsored various smaller groups to help in the resistance of the ACA. In 2009, it launched Patients United Now to warn, via broadcast ads, about government encroachment into health care. It also gave rise to Patients First, which existed for the sake of summer 2009 bus tour of hired speakers to attend rallies and generate opposition to what AfP and its allies often referred to as a "Washington take-over of health care."

The expansion of Medicaid has been an area of particular concern to AfP since the 2012 Supreme Court ruling in *National Federation of Business vs. Sebelius*. The organization has made fighting this a main priority (Roarty 2014). In the many states that wavered on this issue over the past several years, AfP activists have aggressively worked to persuade Republican lawmakers to not give in to organized hospitals' and doctors' associations that have pressed for the expansion. This strategy was largely successful until 2016, at which point several Republican-controlled states reconsidered their initial resistance, with legislators and governors regretting the many millions of federal dollars they were leaving unclaimed by not expanding the program. This slow trickle of Republican states into the expansion category continues to the present, and AfP continues to fight it. A main talking point of the group is that the federal government is an unreliable business partner—language often employed by other oppositional groups—and that state legislators should indeed fear that Congress may not continue funding the Medicaid expansion population at the 90 percent called for in the ACA.

One prominent example of a failed attempt to stop the Medicaid expansion occurred in Virginia in 2018 when AfP ran radio and Facebook ads and organized "Stop Obamacare" meetings in numerous locations in order to dissuade state legislators. AfP staffers bussed hundreds of protestors to the state capitol, dressed them in matching green T-shirts, and provided them with sandwiches from Subway sandwich shop. Despite these efforts, nearly two dozen GOP legislators supported the expansion. Only three of these GOP legislators faced primary election challenges that year (Vozzella 2019). In January 2019, Virginia became the 32nd state to expand Medicaid, albeit with a work requirement that helped make the move more palatable to conservatives.

The Virginia loss notwithstanding, AfP President Tim Phillips has touted the state-by-state strategy as one that he sees as particularly successful. In 2013, he said that "this has been one of those trench warfare kind of efforts for a year now, and I think it is one of those hidden stories of the whole fight against Obamacare. It's not flashy; it's just in a whole bunch of state capitals and in the districts of a whole lot of state legislators, but it's such a critical aspect of the overall long-term effort to roll back Obamacare" (Stolberg 2013). Two years later, still persistent, Phillips commented to a reporter from *The Washington Examiner* newspaper that "from the very beginning, we turned to a state-by-state effort to stop the expansion of Medicaid. Medicaid expansion and Obamacare has been the issue we've worked on more than any other single issue" (Cunningham 2015).

While a precise picture of its finances is not possible, observers have assembled estimates based on IRS reports, AfP publications, and news stories. (501(c)(4) organizations do not have to reveal their contributors, but they must report political contributions.) The expansion since its founding has been dramatic. In 2005, AfP and its fundraising foundation had a budget of some $3.8 million. By 2011, this figure rose to $50 million, and by 2015, it tripled that to reach $150 million (Hertel-Fernandez et al. 2018). AfP spends the large majority of its funds on activities such as sponsoring rallies and the fleets of busses required to deliver the crowds; providing prominent paid speakers for these rallies (Sarah Palin was a favorite for a time); television, radio, and internet ad purchases; and a large paid staff. This reveals a clear preference for mass mobilization, leveraging the free media coverage such events garner, rather than the often tedious work of working alongside law makers to craft public policies. Based on data from the Center for Responsive Politics, in the 2018 election cycle, AfP spent $15.7 million on these outside projects but less than one-half million on traditional lobbying. Its direct contributions to political candidates or campaign committees only amounted to about $16,000.

America's Health Insurance Plans

America's Health Insurance Plans (AHIP) is a prominent Washington, D.C.,-based trade association representing a wide variety of health insurance companies. These firms sell plans on the individual market, through employers, and in the Medicare and Medicaid managed care spaces. AHIP's leadership pursues the expansion of access to affordable health care by way of market-based solutions and policies that provide choice, quality, and innovation and that address high costs. AHIP attracts members, ranging from individuals to large organizations, by sharing industry insights and analytics, facilitating access to policy makers, and fostering contacts that can help insurers sell their products in both the public and private sectors.

AHIP was formed in 2003 by a merger of the Health Insurance Association of America and the American Association of Health Plans. The group underwent significant leadership changes in the 20-teens. Matt Eyles became the president and CEO in 2018. This succession and other significant turnover among senior managers occurred after the association lost three major members: UnitedHealth and Aetna in 2015 and Humana in 2017. These companies' decisions to leave AHIP were partly attributable to a trend involving large health insurers expanding their operations to include medical service delivery. As one example, in 2017 Humana purchased a home health care business, creating an overlap with its Medicare Advantage client base. These large and integrated firms can conduct their own data analytics and have adopted the strategy of hiring their own lobbyists. Given this, paying expensive dues to AHIP came to make less sense for them. Many other insurers are sticking with AHIP, including 12 organizations that joined the association in 2017 (Morse 2018). As of the beginning of 2020, AHIP had 176 member organizations.

The goal of fostering private insurance opportunities and innovation lies at the heart of AHIP's reason for existence. In a September 2019 interview, CEO Matthew Eyles dwelled on several overarching aims for the association (America's Health Insurance Plans 2019b). Discussion of patient-centered care ran through many of his comments. These involve issues of affordability, consumer choice, and the ability of private insurers to closely tailor their products to fit consumer tastes. Envisioning a substantial role for private insurers in both employer-based and government-subsidized programs, such as Medicaid and Medicare managed care, he also spoke about the need to continue making progress toward universal coverage. Eyles emphasized that he thought these goals could be fruitfully pursued in an environment that promotes private-sector innovation. In other words, he favors the practice of government helping individuals to purchase private policies.

In contrast, Eyles opposes Medicare for All, saying that this would not help advance any of the key goals the association prizes and that, unlike what Senator Bernie Sanders (also profiled here) likes to say about a single-payer system, this would not lead to simplicity. Eyles insists that single payer would create longer wait times, worse health outcomes, and higher taxes, and he believes it would represent a clunky government program—akin to "1960s insurance"—without the modern add-ons of Medicare Advantage (Liss 2018). To hear Eyles tell the story, the evolution of Medicare Advantage, again, with its profitable role for private insurers, has converted old-style Medicare into a modern, consumer-friendly form of coverage for its more than 22 million beneficiaries (as of 2019). In other words, in Eyles' view, if Medicare does not continue to work through private insurers, it's retrograde. In support of this position, AHIP co-founded the Partnership for America's Health Care Future in the summer of 2018, which was created to stall any progress by Medicare for All proposals, public options, and other such ideas that would have the federal government become an insurance vendor in direct competition with private insurers.

This critique of the pure government version of Medicare as antiquated and not consumer-friendly does not, however, extend to AHIP's other public messaging about the rest of the ACA. In fact, AHIP wants to defend many provisions of the 2010 law. Recognizing how many customers the ACA has generated for the private insurance industry, AHIP filed an amicus brief in the case of *State of Texas et al. v. United States* after a federal district court judge ruled that the ACA is unconstitutional without the individual mandate, a provision that was rendered inoperative effective January 2019 by way of the federal tax legislation passed in 2017. The U.S. Supreme Court agreed in early 2020 to hear this case. A ruling will likely be delivered by early 2021. To hear the opponents tell the story, the decision depends on whether the justices believe that the individual mandate is severable from the rest of the law. This is a legitimate question, since the drafters of the ACA did not explicitly include a severability clause in the statute's language. There is a history of judges deeming legislatively repealed or constitutionally problematic statutory provisions to be severable even in the absence of explicit severability clauses. In reality, the decision may instead rest on whether a majority of the justices believe this still an ideological battle worth fighting or if instead expanding government health insurance coverage is a train that has already left the station. At stake is no less than whether the entire ACA, with its expansion of both government-based insurance and private coverage, will stand or fall. While the named litigants are the State of Texas and the U.S. Department of Health and Human Services, numerous other states joined in, with predominantly Republican states predictably lining up against the law and predominantly Democratic ones joining in the defense. AHIP's brief argues that to treat the individual mandate as non-severable from the rest of the ACA "would wreak havoc on the health care system" and that "Congress could not have intended that result in 2010" and "did not intend this result in 2017" when it reduced the tax payment to zero for those without insurance (America's Health Insurance Plans 2019a). Indeed, for the ACA to be ruled null and void would be catastrophic for numerous stakeholder groups, including the insurance industry. For the latter, this is not simply an ideological debate, but rather a question of many millions of customers that would be lost.

This recent defense of government activism notwithstanding, over the years AHIP has been what might be considered a reluctant partner. Its predecessor fought the Clinton Plan in the early 1990s with prominently placed television ads designed to sow doubts about the proposal. Obviously, that campaign was successful. However, by the time health care reform was percolating in Congress in 2007 and 2008, AHIP's then CEO, Karen Ignagni, struck a deal with the Obama campaign to not oppose health care reform so long as it included the individual mandate for health insurance (Shaw 2017). AHIP's leadership saw the strong likelihood of health reform passing Congress, and it wanted to help shape that legislation, which meant that spending huge resources opposing it would have been a mistake. As the saying went at the time, for lobbying organizations, it's always better to have a seat at the table than to be on the menu.

Beyond these large questions of government involvement, AHIP has also struggled with the CMS over smaller but still consequential policy issues. For instance, the association recently argued about the calculation of the county-level benchmark prices for Medicare Advantage plans. Specifically, the association argued that this benchmark should be based on the more expensive-to-cover population of people who are eligible for both Part A and Part B, not solely one or the other. As the healthier population with only Part A (the mandatory part of Medicare) grows, the current benchmarking will continue to misrepresent the true price of this population's coverage. As of 2016, 56.5 million are on Part A, compared to only 52.1 million on Part B, which is voluntary. Quibbling about these 4.5 million persons may not seem like much, but the trend is worrisome to profit-seeking insurers that, by design, strive to minimize their financial risks.

Another part of the strategy behind minimizing risk involves private negotiations between insurance companies and the networks of medical providers they contract with when building managed care systems. Neither side wants to conduct these negotiations in public, as they do not want to be seen by their patients or subscribers as profit maximizers. However, this secrecy runs counter to the calls for price transparency that lie at the center of the consumer-driven health care movement, an approach that strives to make health care purchases more like purchases in other economic markets. Here, transparency is fundamental. Thus, when the staff at the CMS, following the requirements written into the ACA, proposed a draft regulation that will require hospitals to publicly list their prices, AHIP and others protested. Insurers say they are worried that consumers will be confused over such lists. In this argument, AHIP has found common cause with the AHA, the Association of American Medical Colleges, the Children's Hospital Association, and the Federation of American Hospitals. These organizations released a joint statement in 2019 claiming that the rule will "introduce widespread confusion, accelerate anti-competitive behavior among health insurers, and stymie innovations in value-based care delivery." The objection says that open pricing will eliminate the opportunity for aggressive bidding by insurance companies and that the net effect will be that prices will go up, not down (Lexology 2019). Depending on one's point of view, this transparency will either make it easier for consumers to shop around or it will undermine competitive negotiations between insurers and employers. AHIP's leadership is adamant that such a rule will limit the extent to which prices can be driven down through negotiations. AHIP's argument lost in federal court in June 2020 (*National Law Review* 2020). As of this writing, the rule will take effect on January 1, 2021.

Despite a rapidly changing health insurance market, it seems likely that AHIP will persist in one form or another for years to come. Its numerous members are certainly willing to bet on this through their organizational dues. The association typically spends much of this income on lobbying. In 2019, AHIP spent just over $7 million on its lobbying activities, more than in any of the previous three years, but less on average per year than it had over the previous decade. Its lobbying expenditures tend to rise and fall with the salience of health care reform initiatives.

Centers for Medicare and Medicaid Services

The CMS is responsible for managing both of these programs, and much more. Administratively, the CMS is housed within the U.S. Department of Health and Human Services, though its headquarters is located near Baltimore, Maryland, where most of its 6,000 staff members are based. It also has regional offices in 10 locations around the country. CMS works with states on Medicare and the Children's Health Insurance Plan. It crafts guidelines for the Health Insurance Portability and Accountability Act (HIPAA). It sets standards for nursing facilities, and it oversees the government's *healthcare.gov* website. CMS is also responsible for developing standards for medical laboratories and for care providers in diverse federal health programs. In order to carry out this work, the CMS issues numerous regulations per year—10,000 pages, give or take—aimed at controlling how taxpayer dollars are spent to consumer safety, to program eligibility and myriad other issues. In many regards, the CMS is the major force in American health care.

Originally named the Bureau of Health Insurance, this agency began at the creation of Medicare and Medicaid. From 1977 to 2001, it was known as the Health Care Financing Administration. As the CMS, it has been responsible for implementing many provisions of the ACA, including the Medicaid expansion, Medicare payment changes. Under the Trump Administration, the agency's politics have been ironic, as the director and her boss have both made a habit of calling for the repeal of the law that they are tasked to enforce and have in fact demonstrated an eagerness to implement in various ways.

The CMS is particularly important in the ways it shapes how objective measures of medical service delivery and outcomes, along with subjective measures of consumer satisfaction, are structured on both the public and private sides of the health sector. For instance, its medical billing codes not only dictate how doctors and hospitals request payments but also influence how for-profit insurers handle billing and the bundling of payments. CMS ways of rating hospitals on service quality have also influenced how private insurers approach contracting with providers in their own networks. Dating back to the early 2000s, CMS, working with the federal Agency for Health Care Research and Quality, developed the Consumer Assessment of Healthcare Providers & Systems (CAHPS) survey. Hospitals that receive payment under Medicare's Inpatient Prospective Payment System must report their quality performance using CAHPS data, covering 32 indicators. While different from the widely used Press Ganey survey of consumer satisfaction, private insurers are mindful of both, and the for-profit Press Ganey organization offers business consulting services to medical providers using the CAHPS assessment tool.

Beyond the day-to-day administration of these large health programs, CMS is a venue for sometimes intense political strategizing and posturing. The agency's administrator is presidentially appointed and senatorially confirmed. Drawing on an Indiana connection provided by Vice President Mike Pence, President Trump appointed Seema Verma to head the agency in 2017. Prior to her government work, she ran a Medicaid consulting business and was a key architect of Indiana's Medicaid expansion, the Healthy Indiana Plan. This plan represents an effort to balance the appeal of broadening Medicaid as part of the ACA with the conservative desire to dress it up as something akin to private insurance through the use of nominal co-payments, monthly premiums, and other steps (Shaw 2017). Taking this strategy forward, Verma has encouraged states to mimic Indiana's approach and to go a step further in allowing state requests to impose work requirements on some Medicaid recipients (though to date these have generally been blocked by courts). For her efforts, Verma has won praise from conservatives for pushing Medicaid and Medicare further toward value-based payments or rewarding providers for delivering quality services. Avik Roy, president of the Foundation for Research on Equal Opportunity, a free-market think tank, said of her that she "has been much more important than in the past in terms of being an engine of policy change" (Meyer 2019). Under her leadership, the CMS has encouraged the expansion of short-term health plans that lack typical consumer protections, and she has spoken out in favor of shifting Medicaid to block grant funding. While advancing these initiatives under Medicaid, Verma has also directly advocated for the repeal of the ACA. As awkward as this disjunction between policy promotion and rhetorical threats may seem, it undoubtedly appeals to Verma's boss.

A couple of controversies stand out in the agency's recent times. One has involved the effort to score hospitals on their quality. In early 2016, the agency proposed a system, called Hospital Compare, under which hospitals can earn up to five stars based on 64 quality metrics. The proposal was widely criticized initially over arguments about methodology and how, in the estimation of the AHA, the system might mislead patients about where they can find quality care. CMS responded by delaying the rollout of this new program, dramatically expanded the range of metrics to be used to over 100, and eventually put it into practice. (Scores and explanations are available at www .medicare.gov/hospitalcompare.) The measures are grouped into seven categories, including mortality, safety of care, readmission, patient experience, effectiveness of care, timeliness of care, and efficient use of medical imaging.

A second issue has garnered many headlines, this one involving Administrator Verma herself. She has used millions of dollars of agency funds to hire Republican-linked media and political consultants to write her speeches and help with public relations. The HHS Office of the Inspector General opened an investigation into whether this spending constituted a violation of agency policy or federal law. As of early 2020, the findings had not been released, due in part to a vacancy at the top of the Office of the Inspector General (Meyer 2019). To leave such watchdog agencies without top administrators has been a common practice under the Trump Administration.

Healthcare-Now!

This Boston-based group was founded in 2004 by the civil rights and health care activist Marilyn Clement (1935–2009). Originally known as the Campaign for a National Health Program NOW, Healthcare-Now! brought together representatives from organized labor, health care, faith-based communities, and others in pursuit of universal government-organized health insurance, specifically a single-payer system. This grassroots organization targets what it characterizes as a fragmented and greedy for-profit insurance industry. The organization holds annual gatherings with advocates, volunteer organizers, and politicians from around the country. These meetings provide opportunities to train grassroots activists. Its 2019 meeting was held in Portland, Oregon.

As an organization chiefly focused on community organizing, some of its consciousness-raising strategies include house parties and street protests. It publishes a protest toolkit on its website (www.healthcare-now.org) to guide grassroots activists. Over the past decade, Healthcare-Now! has coordinated with the California Nurses Association to stage a "National Day of Protest Against Health Insurance Companies," featuring protests in numerous cities in support of a single-payer system. Other direct-action events are regularly discussed in its online quarterly newsletter, *Everybody In!*

On a national level, the organization has supported Senator Bernie Sanders' Healthcare for All Act. In its effort to broaden its political connections, Healthcare-Now! has formed alliances with other organizations that work on national legislation. Its advisory board includes individuals from organized labor, including the United Mine Workers, ideological groups, including the National Organization for Women and Code

Pink, the California Nurses Organization (which is part of National Nurses United), and the prominent public health scholar and single-payer activist David Himmelstein, who co-founded the group Physicians for a National Health Program.

Healthcare-Now! operates an education fund organized as a nonprofit 501(c)(3) organization, which serves as its fundraising vehicle. As a group that is not particularly wealthy, Healthcare-Now! does not focus significant attention on financial contributions to federal candidates.

Kaiser Family Foundation

The Kaiser Family Foundation (KFF) is a highly regarded San Francisco-based nonpartisan think tank that provides policy tracking, analysis, public opinion polling, and skilled journalism on health issues. Its Kaiser Health News unit produces content for print, broadcast, and online news venues. KFF focuses largely on the major government health programs: Medicare, Medicaid, and the ACA. It also partners with public health officials around the country to identify the populations that are most at risk for contracting HIV. Because the organization recognizes that much of its prime audience is in Washington, D.C., KFF maintains an office there as well.

Legally, the Kaiser Family Foundation is a public charity, not a foundation. KFF describes itself as an information organization dedicated to providing high-quality information about America's $3 trillion health care system. In recognizing that the government is such a major player in the health care sector, KFF extensively focuses its work on public policy. Its policy tracking and analysis allows a wide variety of stakeholders and observers—including researchers, government officials, journalists, and ordinary American—to stay abreast of the latest developments in program use, the impact of government regulations, and many other issues. The information contained in its reports (many of which are relied on as sources for the chapters of this book) are useful for both expert and lay audiences.

Their policy tracking work on Medicare, Medicaid, and to a lesser extent the private insurance markets allows readers to keep up on the current developments. Since the passage of the ACA in particular, KFF has become a primary source for nonpartisan information on the Medicaid expansion in the states and on public opinion toward the ACA and its various components. The KFF polling unit has partnered with the Harvard School of Public Health and with journalists at National Public Radio and *The Washington Post*. KFF strives to be a trusted force to enhance public debate. They do not take positions on policy proposals.

The KFF was established in 1948 by Henry J. Kaiser, the early-20th century industrialist, philanthropist, and founder of Kaiser Permanente, the health management company. Since 1985, the Kaiser Family Foundation has not had a relationship with Kaiser Permanente. KFF is guided by a board of trustees, currently chaired by Jim Doyle, former governor of Wisconsin. Its president, Drew Altman, is a widely recognized expert on health policy who previously worked at the Pew Center for the People and the Press and the Robert Wood Johnson Foundation. Most of the KFF's annual funding comes from an endowment and the remainder from contributions from philanthropic foundations and the numerous local public health departments that partner with KFF on HIV/AIDS research and education as part of the Greater Than AIDS project. Its current funders include the Bill and Melinda Gates Foundation, the American Association of Retired Persons, Walgreens, the media company Viacom, and various foundations.

The Kaiser Family Foundation is particularly visible in its tracking of public opinion on the ACA. Its monthly Health Tracking Poll began in the months just prior to the passage of the ACA. This longitudinal study became the definitive measure of public opinion and public knowledge about the ACA from 2010 forward. By asking many of the same questions over time, the Health Tracking Poll allowed experts and generalists alike to gain a better understanding of what parts of the controversial law were gaining or losing in the way of public approval, how those sentiments varied by demographic characteristics and political party identification, and what the public actually understood about the law. Interactive graphics at the KFF website (www.kff.org) allow users to parse polling data in various ways. In addition to its polling work, the KFF has tracked developments in the Medicaid expansion and demographic trends among the still-uninsured population. It also routinely publishes reports on Medicare Advantage policy developments, health care spending, trends among employer-based insurance arrangements, and many other health-related topics.

On the journalism side, KFF started the editorially independent *Kaiser Health News* in 2009. The goal is to produce quality coverage of the complex topics of health care that go beyond what commercial news outlets can or will provide. Kaiser Health News is now the largest health policy newsroom in the country, providing content for print, broadcast, and online venues. KFF works with a wide variety of national news outlets, public health departments, and other entities to disseminate information about health care and health policy. In recognizing KFF in 2018, the American Medical Associate presented it with the Outstanding Government Service Award. The then president of the AMA, Dr. Nathan David, commended the KFF for its contributions to public discourse on health issues, noting that it "served a key role during the 2017 congressional debate on the ACA, providing data-driven analyses, studies and surveys about the impact of the proposed House and Senate reform bills. The Foundation hosted a range of ACA studies on its website, including a recent 50-state survey about the future of Medicaid and a tool to help patients calculate their 2018 ACA premiums and tax credits" (American Medical Association 2018). The foundation has done impressive work to provide materials that inform the public discourse on health issues. Whether partisan politicians and their followers choose to use this information is, of course, another issue.

National Nurses United

National Nurses United was founded in 2009 as a means to give political voice to registered nurses and other patient care staff. In recent years, it has operated mainly as a labor union for nurses and as a grassroots advocacy organization that has spent much of its energy and fundraising capacity to call for Medicare for All. Based in Silver Spring, Maryland, this organization was created by the merger of the California Nurses Association, the National Nurses Organizing Committee, the United American Nurses, and the Massachusetts Nurses Association. National Nurses United is the largest nurse association in the United States, with more than 150,000 members in 22 states. Its director, Bonnie Castillo, is a registered nurse. Reflecting its labor union imprimatur and unapologetic focus on progressive politics, the organization is an affiliate of the AFL/CIO. Unlike the older and less overtly political American Nurses Association, National Nurses United has not shied away from wading into the controversial advocacy of single-payer health care financing. This stance is driven in large part by the perspective Castillo takes that sees nursing as a field of service that goes beyond treating patients' physiological problems in clinical settings. She wants her organization to fight for a larger set of considerations relating to the social and economic well-being of patients. Her slogan "vote nurses' values" is intended to capture a broad swath of concerns, ranging from the economic vulnerability of the uninsured to discrimination along the lines of sexual orientation and race, to union representation more generally (Castillo 2019).

National Nurses United has been particularly visible over the past few years as an organizing body for street-level protests for Medicare for All and has intentionally targeted the offices of some organizations it sees as foes, including PhRMA, the U.S. Chamber of Commerce, and big Wall Street banks. The organization also endorsed Bernie Sanders for president in 2019. Jasmine Ruddy, the organization's coordinator of its campaign for Medicare for All, characterizes universal health care access as a human right. In a June 2019 interview, she noted that nurses are the caregivers who sit in rooms with patients who are often forced to choose between paying their rent and for groceries on one hand and their health care on the other. She went on to emphasize that "the root of the problem is the private insurance industry. And Medicare for All is the only solution that gets rid of that . . . We're talking about getting rid of the insurance companies and changing the way we pay for services" (Darby 2019). This idea picks up on Sanders' proposal to make Medicare the payer for all Americans and that his bill would prohibit private insurers from covering services that Medicare covers. In the U.S. House of Representatives, Pramila Jayapal of Seattle, Washington, has introduced a bill (H.R. 1384) that is a variation on the Sanders bill. If enacted, this legislation would relegate whatever remnants of the private insurance industry that survived to a minor role in health care financing.

Executive Director Castillo shares the enthusiasm for a single-payer solution. Speaking at a rally called to mark Representative Jayapal's February 2019 introduction of her version of Medicare for All, Castillo said that "we could not be more proud of [Representative] Jayapal for leading the way on this legislation that will change and save our patients' lives. This bill is not only the most comprehensive Medicare for All act we have seen to date, but it is being introduced at a time when a majority of Americans are fed up with incremental tweaks to the current broken system and are demanding Medicare for All" (National Nurses United 2019).

In order to amplify the movement from scattered protests and relatively modest contributions to congressional candidates to something larger, National Nurses United conducted door-to-door canvassing in some 1,500 locations in 2019 (Darby 2019). While the organization has focused its campaign contributions on Democrats, organizer Ruddy understands that they will also need Republican support. She notes that advocates will need to organize working-class people in Red states and districts as well and that they believe it is possible to frame universal health care access as an issue with broad appeal. Of course, recent evidence on support for and opposition to the ACA clearly indicates this is much easier said than done.

During the 2018 federal election cycle, National Nurses United made direct contributions to 43 U.S. House candidates, all Democrats, and to two U.S. Senate candidates, Bernie Sanders of Vermont and Kevin de Leon of California, who unsuccessfully challenged incumbent Senator Dianne Feinstein. Its finances are modest compared to the other organizations profiled here. In the 2018 election cycle, it received total contributions of $590,000 and spent $680,000.

Partnership for America's Health Care Future

This consortium was created in the summer of 2018 with the specific goal of derailing calls for Medicare for All. The Partnership consists of health insurers and their main lobbying group, AHIP, together with local and state chambers of commerce, the Pharmaceutical Research and Manufacturers of America (PhRMA), the AHA, the Blue Cross Blue Shield Association, and others. The group has particularly focused on dissuading moderate Democrats from what these opponents fear could become a broadly embraced idea on the political Left. Seeking to turn back a range of possible proposals for greater government health insurance, this group's messaging treats the terms Medicare for All, Medicare buy-in, and a public option as equivalents. Its strategy is to undermine support for universal Medicare before this notion can evolve from being a merely aspirational idea among progressive Democrats into a major plank in the party's platform. This organization presents itself as a moderate voice in support of existing programs, including the ACA's Medicaid expansion. Its central message is that Americans should stick with what works well in the combination of public and private health insurance and to not endanger existing programs through efforts to start something new.

The Partnership pursues a decentralized communications strategy. Instead of hiring its own lobbyists to pressure members of Congress, it works mainly through its member organizations both at the state level and in the nation's capital to push messaging about how the existing combination of Medicare, Medicaid, employer-based insurance, and the online Marketplace established under the ACA serves Americans well. Its members spent an estimated $143 million on lobbying in 2018 (Stein 2019). Typical of the messaging is a comment from Charles Kahn III, the president of the Federation of American Hospitals, who said that any health policy reforms should be made to "work for all Americans. We reject the notion that we need to turn the whole apple cart over and start all over again" (Pear 2019). Of course, starting over is exactly what Bernie Sanders' plan envisions. If enacted, the Sanders plan would preclude private insurers covering health services already included in Medicare. Potentially private insurers could find a niche in specialty services, experimental treatments, and the likes to prop up their businesses, though this dramatically diminished service sector would almost certainly spell the demise of most of the present private insurance industry.

The Partnership's executive director, Lauren Crawford Shaver, previously worked for Hillary Clinton's 2016 campaign. Shaver succeeded in recruiting more than two dozen affiliates during 2018 and 2019, including the AMA and the AHA, two organizations that have been beneficiaries of the influx of paying customers created by the ACA. Despite this assistance, these groups harbor deep concerns about a potentially new environment in which their patient mix would tilt strongly toward Medicare and its money-losing levels of reimbursements to medical providers. Despite this broad coalition building, the leadership of the AMA in summer 2019 made news by pulling out of the project, with its CEO James Madera issuing a statement to the effect that while the nation's largest doctors' association shares deep concerns about a single-payer health system, it wants to focus on practical solutions for the millions of Americans who still lack health insurance (Luthi 2019; Sullivan 2019).

Forbes Tate, a public affairs company that lobbies for many health care and drug companies, coordinates the work of the Partnership, but it's not registered to lobby on its behalf. To date, the strategy has been to generate studies that they can disseminate among think tanks, journalists, politicians, and others designed to emphasize how expensive Medicare for All would be and how health services would, they believe, inevitably decline in quality. The organization has distributed fliers to Democratic congressional staffers, warning of the dangers of a public option plan or Medicare for All (Stein 2019). The Partnership emphasizes what it says would create a loss of control for consumers, as the nearly 180 million Americans who currently enjoy insurance through employers would be forced to trade in that coverage for a government-run plan that the Partnership characterizes as bureaucratically inefficient and controlled by politicians. The epithet "one-size-fits-all" features prominently in its online messaging as a way of characterizing this new world of government health insurance.

In addition to the idea of a health care system hobbled by bureaucracy, the Partnership also makes much of the high costs of Medicare for All. Following the lead of the Congressional Budget Office and its projected $32 trillion price tag for the first decade of the Sanders plan (S 1129), the Partnership raises the alarm that paying for this would mean a doubling of the average American's income tax liability. (The Urban Institute produced a similar price estimate.) In their materials, there is no mention of how much this shift would save employers and, in turn, their employees. Instead, the message is that tax experts insist that taxing the rich—a mainstay of some progressive Democrats' rhetoric—would be insufficient to pay for Medicare for All. The emphasis when discussing the finances of this idea is overwhelmingly focused on what it would cost taxpayers, not on the fact that insurance companies would face an existential threat under such legislation. Of course, such a commentary would not likely carry much water, given the low esteem in which many Americans hold insurers.

In contrast, Americans generally hold positive attitudes toward their medical providers, and this theme also figures prominently in the Partnership's online messaging. Readers find there a variety of warnings about how devastating Medicare for All would be for hospitals. A source quoted in a September 2019 *New York Times* article warned of "violent upheaval" that would accompany a Medicare for All system, causing "some hospitals, especially struggling rural centers, [to] close virtually overnight . . . Others . . . would try to offset the steep cuts by laying off hundreds of thousands of workers and abandoning lower-paying services like mental health" (Abelson 2019).

As an industry group representing insurers, pharmaceutical companies, and hospital groups, the Partnership for America's Health Care Future predictably supports the status quo, given how over the past decade these groups have benefitted tremendously by the influx of paying customers, newly covered by the ACA. Of course, these groups still rely on a mix of private-pay customers to subsidize the low-pay Medicare and Medicaid patients they treat, and for this reason, the Partnership opposes a radical shift in this patient mix. As of this writing, it is difficult to judge the near-term prospects for a Medicare for All proposal, be it the bill sponsored by Vermont Senator Bernie Sanders or some other version. However, it seems improbable that any such bill could make its way through the U.S. Senate lacking the supermajority of Democrats in play during the 2010 passage of the ACA.

Pharmaceutical Research and Manufacturers of America

PhRMA is the main lobbying organization for the U.S. biopharmaceutical industry. Based in Washington, D.C., PhRMA also has offices in Japan and the United Arab Emirates. Formed in 1958 and originally called the Pharmaceutical Manufacturers

Association, PhRMA is a 501(c)(3) nonprofit organization, which means it can operate on a tax-free basis, though it must publicly report its donors, unlike some other types of pressure groups. As a federally registered lobbying group, it is active in the nation's capital, but it also works in states on such concerns as ballot measures and electoral campaigns that might affect the drug industry. In recent years, PhRMA has represented between 35 and 50 pharmaceutical companies. The organization says it focuses its work in three areas: patient access to effective medicines through market-based solutions that do not involve government price controls, strong protection of intellectual property rights, and transparent and effective regulation involving a free flow of information to patients. In line with this philosophy, PhRMA tends to maintain strong ties to Republican office holders.

Over the past two decades, PhRMA has found itself in the news particularly over two key issues. The first was the 2003 passage of the Medicare Modernization Act and what is widely regarded as a sweetheart deal written into the noninterference clause of that statute. As discussed in Chapter 2, this clause prohibits the Secretary of the Department of Health and Human Services from interfering with price negotiations between insurance companies and drug manufacturers that participate in Medicare's Part D (Shih et al. 2016). This means that Medicare cannot use its bulk purchasing power to negotiate lower drug prices. The story of how PhRMA's then head, Billy Tauzin, helped shepherd this deal through Congress has been documented in numerous journalistic and academic venues (Oliver et al. 2004; Aaron and Lambrew 2008; Potter and Penniman 2016). This inhibition has been the source of consternation for many members of Congress, particularly Democrats, and has been targeted by a proposed legislation, including a 2019 bill aimed at overturning the rule (Pollack 2015).

Second, PhRMA has found itself on the receiving end of numerous attacks over steeply rising retail drug prices in recent years. The accusation usually takes the form that the lobbying group is more interested in defending its profit-seeking members than it is in helping ordinary Americans to afford their prescriptions. While this a more complex issue than can be settled here, it is certainly true that PhRMA has lobbied Congress to preserve its members' ability to price their drugs in ways that have little, if anything, to do with the actual costs of development, manufacturing, and distribution. The instances of drug companies purchasing a patent and subsequently increasing the retail price of their newly acquired drug by ten-fold or more are numerous (Alpern et al. 2014; Angell 2015; Bach 2016).

Much of the political debate over pharmaceutical pricing has turned on sales under Part D, given that this line of programming accounts for most of Medicare's drug spending. This amounted to $99.5 billion in 2016 (Kaiser Family Foundation 2016). Given how important this is, PhRMA has spent a great deal of energy engaging policy makers. Of course, a large part of this effort has gone into defending the Medicare Modernization Act's noninterference clause. This is a fight many Democrats would relish, and House Speaker Nancy Pelosi sponsored a bill that would repeal this provision. Beyond this, however, several other arguably second-tier but still consequential issues have garnered attention in recent years.

First, there is the matter of how drug makers are incentivized to price their products. Under the current rules, pharmaceutical manufacturers set a price list for each of their drugs. At the pharmacy counter, customers pay co-payments and deductibles based on their Part D benefit plan, and their insurance company pays the remainder. However, behind the curtain where these prices are set, a group of actors called pharmacy benefit managers negotiate with drug makers over which drugs will be included in which benefit plans. These lists, or formularies, directly affect the sales volume of drugs. This practice is to credit for helping boost the sales of generic drugs, for instance. However, because pharmacy benefit managers—who often contract to work as intermediaries between drug makers and insurance companies—currently receive kickbacks from drug makers in exchange for placing their products on formularies, drug makers face an incentive to raise their prices in order to compensate for the expense of the kickbacks, sometimes called rebates (Antos and Capretta 2019). This is similar to food manufacturers paying supermarkets for prime shelf placements of their products. In pursuit of President Trump's stated goal of reducing retail drug prices, in the spring of 2019, the Administration proposed a draft rule that would have curtailed this practice (Roy 2019). This would have allowed the president to claim credit for eliminating this layer of middlemen. (There is debate about whether or not this move would have actually saved money for seniors.) However, strong resistance during the summer of 2019 from the organized interests that own these pharmacy benefit manager operations led to an abrupt dropping of the proposed rule, with the White House saying it wanted Congress to develop a solution to the problem. In the wake of this reversal, the major pharmacy benefit management firms, including Cigna Express Scripts, CVS Health Caremark, and UnitedHealth Group's Optum Rx, all saw their stock prices rise significantly that week (Japsen 2019b). For its part, PhRMA, which favored the change, lamented the administration's decision to withdraw the rule, calling it "a blow to seniors who could have paid less for their medicines at the pharmacy counter" (Porter 2019).

In another recent loss, PhRMA has worked to foster a repeal of the ACA. The law's various provisions aimed at curtailing overall health spending represents a problem, particularly the fees imposed on drug makers. However, the organization has not always waged a frontal assault on the ACA, likely because its leadership realizes Americans' growing acceptance of and in many cases reliance on its benefits. In early 2017, when congressional Republicans and the Trump Administration were gearing up to attempt a repeal of the ACA, PhRMA publicly stated its neutrality. However, at the same time the group was quietly diverting millions of dollars to the conservative American Action Network, a 501(c)(4) organization that is not required to reveal its donors and which purchased an advertisement campaign designed to build voter support for repealing the ACA (*Axos* 2018; Hancock 2018). The persuasion campaign involved radio and television ads as well as robocalls placed numerous times in 75 congressional districts. PhRMA's contributions came to light only later, when it was required to report its spending to the federal government. PhRMA contributions to the American Action Network during 2017 amounted to $6.1 million. While this did not result in the ACA's repeal, it certainly begins to illustrate PhRMA's determination.

Spending $6 million on this ad campaign would seem like a great deal for most health care lobbying organizations, but PhRMA is well endowed. Between 2010 and 2014, its annual revenue ranged from $200 to $205 million. During 2017, it spent $128 million on lobbying.

Physicians for a National Health Program

This progressive organization supports a single-payer health care system and represents over 23,000 members nationwide. Based in Chicago, this organization was founded in 1987 by the practicing physicians and public health scholars Steffie Woolhander and David Himmelstein. The organization supports research into the consequences of being without health insurance, and it works to educate fellow physicians and the public on these issues. They support the proposed Medicare for All Act of 2019, Senator Bernie Sanders bill (S. 1129). Specifically, they want to see the elimination of point-of-service co-payments and deductibles, to limit the duration of drug patents in order to speed medicines to the generic market more quickly than is currently the practice, and they advocate for extending health insurance to all Americans, regardless of immigration status.

The organization's frequent press releases are a key part of its communications strategy. As one example, in October 2019 it sought to amplify a Harvard Medical School study that appeared that month in the *American Journal of Public Health*. The researchers present analysis suggesting that extending health insurance to all would not likely lead to the explosive growth in service utilization—due to what economists call moral hazard—in the health care sector. For instance, prior to the passage of Medicare and Medicaid in 1965, Americans averaged 427 doctor visits and 7 surgical procedures per 100 persons annually. After these programs were put in place, these figures remained essentially unchanged, at 425 visits and 7 procedures per 100 persons annually. Following the implementation of the ACA, the comparable figures for 2014 were 327 doctor visits and 16 procedures per 100 persons annually. The study also found no shortage in access to providers or care shortages. Because these concerns are important parts of the argument against Medicare for All, this evidence is very much in line with what the organization wants to disseminate. Of course, other concerns about single-payer, whether those are philosophical or about taxes, lie beyond the scope of this kind of research.

Physicians for a National Health Program also organizes direct action in the form of street protests. One such event occurred in November 2019 in Philadelphia when more than 100 doctors, medical students, and other advocates gathered downtown to demand that the U.S. House Representative, Dwight Evans (D), support H.R. 1384, the Medicare for All Act. At the time, this bill had 118 House sponsors, including a majority of the Democratic House caucus. Speakers at the event noted that the council of the City of Philadelphia had recently adopted a resolution supporting single-payer, bolstering the idea that Representative Evans faces significant pressure to co-sponsor the bill (Physicians for a National Health Program 2019).

Another street protest was organized in Chicago in the summer of 2019 at the headquarters of the insurer Blue Cross/Blue Shield. From there, the protesters marched to the site of the annual meeting of the AMA to call attention to the claim that most American physicians support single-payer and that the time was right for the AMA's leadership to leave the anti-Medicare for All group, the Partnership for America's Health Care Future, a move that the AMA indeed took later that summer.

As what might be considered a shoe-string operation, Physicians for a National Health Program does not have a fundraising profile that rises to the level of triggering federal reporting under the Lobbying Disclosure Act. Its media-based communications strategies and street-level pressure tactics do not require formal registration as a federal lobbying group.

Senator Bernie Sanders (b. September 8, 1941)

U.S. Senator Bernie Sanders of Vermont (formally an Independent, but he caucuses with Democrats) has done more than any other national politician to shift the terms of discussion of a single-payer health system among Democrats over the past decade. He has introduced multiple bills in Congress to create a single-payer system, an idea that has been generally referred to as Medicare for All since about 2015. While the bills he has introduced have not made any real progress through the labyrinthine legislative process, his rhetorical advocacy for universal health care as a basic human right has convinced many on the political Left to embrace this idea, where they saw it as too risky only a few years earlier. Whereas he was the only candidate in the Democratic field in 2016 to call for Medicare for All, several of the 2020 Democratic candidates fell in line with him on this issue, at least initially. Regardless of how this issue plays out over the next few election cycles, observers will credit Sanders for transforming a fringe idea into one that has gained a mainstream following.

Sanders has made universal health care a centerpiece of his work in Congress and his campaign rhetoric. The position he staked out fits well with his progressive populist identity. He has built a substantial following by demonizing the private health insurance and pharmaceutical industries. He routinely accuses these two groups of robbing Americans of billions of dollars each year, and he relishes the prospect of essentially doing away with private insurance and of limiting drug company profits through a combination of price limits and government negotiation over drug prices.

During the 116th Congress, Sanders introduced Senate bill 1129, the Medicare for All Act of 2019. Upon its introduction, he secured the support of 14 cosponsors, including 2020 presidential candidates Elizabeth Warren (D-MA), Cory Booker (D-NJ), Kamala Harris (D-CA), and Kirsten Gillibrand (D-NY). While some of these candidates gradually distanced themselves from Sanders' plan as the campaign season progressed, the idea became a main reference point for many politicians in the Democratic Party. Debate moderators routinely asked candidates if they support Sanders' ideas. The 2019 bill would extend Medicare to cover all U.S. residents, regardless of immigration status. Sanders touts this as a program that would eliminate all fees at the point of service, meaning no deductibles, no co-payments, no surprise bills, and no separate premiums. It remains unclear exactly how the program would be paid for, but the general idea is that instead of Americans paying hundreds of billions of dollars to private health insurers each year, they would pay some portion of those dollars to the federal government, which would then operate this expanded version of Medicare in a more efficient way, free of the need to earn a profit. Sanders' expanded version of Medicare would cover dental, hearing, vision, home and community-based long-term care, inpatient and outpatient care, mental health, substance abuse treatment, reproductive and maternity care, prescription drugs.

One of the more controversial—and less broadly supported—ideas in the Sanders bill is that it would prohibit the sale of private insurance that would duplicate Medicare coverage. Publicly Sanders has referred to whatever remnant of the private insurance industry that might persist as something that could cover such services as cosmetic surgery. Of course, there is no insurance market for such services—no one buys insurance because they are considering getting their nose fixed—so Sanders' rhetoric on this point can, arguably, be understood as an artful dodge around what is for some the uncomfortable prospect of losing the private insurance policy that they have and like. Further illustrating the ambition of the Sanders plan, it is noteworthy that this system would be more comprehensive than single-payer plans in other developed nations, and more so than the plan briefly adopted by his home state of Vermont. For instance, it is common for Western European health systems to use general practitioners as gatekeepers that limit patient access specialists as a cost-saving move. Further, co-payments are common in single-payer systems, whereas the Sanders plan would eliminate them.

A particular target of Sanders' rhetoric is the pharmaceutical industry. He says his plan would "stop the pharmaceutical industry from ripping off the American people by making sure that no one in America pays over $200 per year for the medicine they need by capping" prices under Medicare for All. He points out that high medical bills are the primary reason for personal bankruptcies in the United States. Among other changes, Sanders wants to allow Medicare to negotiate prices with drug companies and to import drugs from Canada, a change that the Trump Administration supported in a Food and Drug Administration rule change proposed in December 2019. This proposal remains in limbo as of the spring of 2020, particularly because the main pharmacy distribution companies in Canada are not eager to participate, given the frequent supply shortages in that country.

The other chief target of Sanders' plan is the private insurance industry. He routinely calls out insurers on what he says is their greed. In April 2019, he targeted UnitedHealth (also profiled here), saying "your greed is going to end" (Armstrong and Tozzi 2019). Part of the craving he had in mind speaks to a lawsuit that claims that UnitedHealth systematically shook down Medicare by raising the risk-adjustment scores of Medicare Advantage plan enrollees by retrospectively reviewing medical records and searching for additional diagnoses, which had the effect of pulling down millions of dollars more than its subsidiary OptumInsight arguably deserved. Insurers participating in Medicare Advantage have an incentive to identify every complicating diagnosis of their covered persons. More complicated diagnoses lead to high risk-adjustment scores, which lead to larger government payments. The U.S. Department of Justice joined the suit in early 2017 (Livingston 2018).

The 2019 version of the Sanders plan would provide broad coverage for all residents of the United States, regardless of income and immigration status. Several large issues remain unsettled. One has to do with payment levels to providers. Since a shrinking percentage of doctors' offices are unwilling to accept Medicaid in recent years, would the Sanders' version of Medicare for All avoid this problem? Another major question is about how to pay for the plan. Based on a couple of thoughtful analyses (including one by the Urban Institute—see Chapter 2 for discussion), this would cost in the neighborhood of $32 trillion over its first decade. Of course, Sanders insists that this is less than Americans will likely pay to their private insurers during this period, though this large price tag still makes his plan a hard sell. The Sanders camp had advanced a series of potential funding sources—essentially new taxes—that could raise the necessary funds in ways that fit with his political outlook. On his website in early 2020, he listed the following:

- Creating a 4 percent income-based premium paid by employees, exempting the first $29,000 in income for a family of four
- Imposing a 7.5 percent income-based premium paid by employers, exempting the first $2 million in payroll
- Eliminating health tax expenditures

- Making the federal income tax more progressive, including a marginal tax rate of up to 70 percent on those making above $10 million
- Making the estate tax more progressive, including a 77 percent top rate on an inheritance above $1 billion
- Establishing a tax on extreme wealth
- Closing a tax loophole that allows self-employed people to avoid paying certain taxes by creating an S corporation
- Imposing a fee on large financial institutions

Skeptics point out that Vermont attempted to create a single-payer system in 2014, and this turned out to be unsuccessful. That plan was less ambitious than the Sanders Medicare for All bill. For instance, the Vermont plan required patients to make co-payments at the point of service. Vermont's single-payer plan lost support once state policy makers got a realistic sense of how expensive it would be and that the required tax increases were politically unpopular, specifically, payroll taxes by 11.5 percent and income tax by 9 percent (Kliff 2016).

In the months leading up to the 2020 presidential primary election season, Sanders temporarily gained a prominent ally in his cause for single payer in Massachusetts Senator and fellow Democratic presidential hopeful Elizabeth Warren. In late 2019, in what might be seen as a pragmatic move to position herself a bit closer to the ideological center, Warren shifted away from her call for an abrupt move to Medicare for All and instead suggested that a public insurance option could serve as an interim step toward single payer. True to his belief, Sanders didn't budge. Even in suspending his presidential campaign in April 2020, Sanders stubbornly insisted that he was proud of having shifted the terms of debate over health care in America. Regardless of what one thinks of Sanders' unapologetic stances, it is clear from public opinion polling that Sanders has played a part in moving many Democrats toward a single-payer approach to health insurance.

UnitedHealth Group, Inc.

UnitedHealth Group is the world's largest health insurer. Based in Minnetonka, Minnesota, and employing some 300,000 workers, it sells insurance plans through its two subsidiaries, UnitedHealthcare, and Optum, plus a variety of affiliates organized on state-by-state and regional bases. In addition to its insurance businesses, UnitedHealth Group also operates a series of outpatient care centers, a data analytics operation, and a large pharmacy benefit management business. This diversity enhances its profitability. UnitedHealth's share price increased ten-fold between the bottom of the Great Depression and the autumn of 2019. The companies in the group have benefitted tremendously by changes under the ACA, specifically the large influx of new subscribers (Ward 2019). In 2018, UnitedHealth Group had revenue of $226 billion, and it serviced some 115 million customers, nearly as many as Medicare itself (Business Wire 2019). Servicing the managed care elements of Medicare and Medicaid make up a large part of UnitedHealth's business.

The exposure that UnitedHealth has in the Medicare and Medicaid managed care markets makes its leadership highly attuned to possible reforms to those programs. Like several other large stakeholders described in this chapter, United-Health has found ways to work with and alongside government-backed health insurance while simultaneously preferring that the federal and state governments do not enlarge their footprints in these markets. The financial and political balancing act involved here led UnitedHealth to maintain a somewhat low profile about talk of expanding Medicare over the past several years. However, as Senator Bernie Sanders and other presidential candidates amplified their advocacy of this in the spring of 2019, the company's leaders in turn became more strident in their opposition. Up to that point, by its own description, the company tried to maintain a low profile, though in the words of one of their executives, Steve Nelson, "you want to be kind of thoughtful about how you show up and have these kind of conversations, because the last thing you want to do is become a poster child during the presidential campaign" (Stein 2019). The company wanted to avoid becoming the target of a powerful campaign by a leading presidential candidate, in the way that PhRMA experienced. However, as the perceived credibility of calls for Medicare for All grew, UnitedHealth's spokespersons grew more vigorous in their pushback. The company joined the Partnership for America's Health Care Future in the summer of 2018, and its public statements during 2019 became increasingly blunt. Dave Wichmann, the CEO of UnitedHealth Group, stated in early 2019 that a shift to Medicare for All would amount to a "wholesale disruption of American health care" (Armstrong and Tozzi 2019). Of course, for their part, supporters of Medicare for All explicitly want to disrupt what they see as wasteful profit-taking at the expense of ordinary Americans.

UnitedHealth Group PAC functions as the company's political action committee. The PAC annually publishes a transparent report of its political advocacy, which is available online. It states that its central mission is to help develop solutions to deliver health insurance to all Americans in a high-quality and long-term sustainable way that lowers costs. While it prefers to pursue market-based solutions, the PAC financially supports candidates, office holders, and fundraising committees in both political parties. Casting a broad net, it also strives to work with policy makers at the local, state, and federal levels. The strategy at work here is nothing if not pragmatic. The PAC is willing to work with a wide variety of actors. This extends to other advocacy entities, from which the UnitedHealth Group PAC regularly receives contributions. In 2018, this list of groups included the U.S. Chamber of Commerce, various medical lobbying groups, several private insurers and insurance plan administrators, the American College of Physicians, and the American Academy of Actuaries, among many others. More than two dozen groups contributed in excess of $50,000 each during 2018 (UnitedHealth Group PAC 2019). The PAC used these funds to support a wide variety of office holders, including direct donations to both Democrats and Republicans in Congress, as well as several leadership PACs organized by members of Congress. UnitedHealth Group PAC also donated $15,000 each to the Democratic Congressional Campaign Committee and the Republican National Campaign Committee in 2018. In addition to its direct contributions, the PAC also engages in extensive lobbying activities, which amounted to $4.1 million during 2018. This was less than the $4.8 million it spent in 2017 but more than it spent during most years since the passage of the ACA.

U.S. Chamber of Commerce

The U.S. Chamber of Commerce is the highest spending lobbying and political pressure group in the United States. Based in Washington, D.C., it raises funds from its thousands of members and spends many millions of dollars each year lobbying both federal and state governments on a wide variety of concerns. Beyond lobbying Congress and the executive branch, the Chamber makes sizable financial contributions to federal candidates, files amicus briefs to the federal courts, and funds public education and persuasion campaigns, among other pressure tactics.

The U.S. Chamber of Commerce was founded at a gathering of business leaders in 1912. President Taft encouraged its creation as counter-balance to the growing labor unions of the time. The organization grew rapidly during the 19-teens, reaching over 300 within its first decade. The organization's staff currently numbers over 400. In line with its founding purpose, the Chamber has strongly tended to support market-based approaches to health care spending and delivery problems. However, in a move that was not quite in keeping with this posture, the Chamber supported the Clinton health plan in the early 1990s, recognizing that action was needed in order to confront steeply rising costs, a burden that affected not only families and governments but also employers. However, since then the Chamber has stuck mainly to pro-market positions and remains opposed to greater government involvement in health care financing and delivery. It supported the passage of the Medicare Modernization Act in 2003, though, judging from its communications at the time, it did so in large part to promote and support the hundreds of thousands of Americans who make their living in the pharmaceutical industry, a sector that was in for a major boost as the new drug benefit spread across the Medicare population.

In recent years, the U.S. Chamber of Commerce has enjoyed gross annual revenues in excess of $100 million. In 2018, the Chamber spent over $94 million on lobbying, far more than any other single group (Center for Responsive Politics 2020). Since the mid-2000s, its spending has focused particularly on federal candidates, exceeding $100 million in several elections. This organization typically directs the vast majority of its spending to Republican candidates. During the 2020 election cycle, Senate Majority Leader Mitch McConnell has easily been its top recipient.

Regarding health care, the Chamber takes the position that promoting effective private-sector solutions is preferable to government controls on markets or government mandates aimed at employers. Reflecting its membership of business firms, it maintains a strong focus on employer-based insurance as a platform that is controllable by private companies and that is often used as a recruiting tool. Leaving such choices in employers' hands instead of with government allows businesses to closely tailor their benefit packages in ways that reflect their priorities and local market conditions, quite the opposite of any notion of standardized benefits required by government. Not only does the Chamber oppose mandates for employers to provide any particular kind of health coverage, but it also stands for the right of employers to decline to provide insurance at all if the employer would prefer not to do so.

Reflecting this commitment to employer autonomy, in 2001 the Chamber's affiliated Institute for Legal Reform staked out a position in opposition to the Kennedy-McCain Patient's Bill of Rights because its leadership feared this would open the door to excessive litigation that would cost employers too much (U.S. Chamber of Commerce 2001). Tracing that philosophy forward in time, over the past decade the Chamber has taken the position that the ACA, with its Medicaid expansion and heightened Medicare regulation, should be repealed. The Chamber filed amicus briefs both in the 2011 cases of *National Federation of Independent Businesses v. Sebelius*, having to do with the Medicaid expansion and the individual mandate to purchase insurance, as well as the latter case of *King v. Burwell*, which had mainly to do with federal subsidies to individuals who purchase insurance on the federal *healthcare.gov* Marketplace. In its court documents, the Chamber says that the ACA should be repealed because of the rising costs the act imposes on employers, and it particularly opposes the medical device tax, the Cadillac tax, and the employer mandate. In late 2019, as part of a larger spending agreement that won bipartisan support, Congress repealed the medical device tax and the Cadillac tax.

In what might be considered a desire to have it both ways, the Chamber in 2018 took the position that it wanted Medicare to be the primary insurance for retirees who also have a group policy provided by a former employer. Depending on the nature of the group plan, the size of the employer's workforce, and other factors, Medicare is sometimes designated as a secondary payer, meaning the former employer's plan must pay first, a rule that the Chamber opposes, along with, presumably, most of its members. Hence, while the Chamber touts its market-based solutions most of the time, instances such as this illustrate a desire to save member employers' money by asking the federal government to pay most of the bills. Striking a similar position, the Chamber also argues that employers should be able to fund retirees' health insurance on a tax-preferred basis just as they do when funding the health insurance premiums for their current workers. Under current law (as of 2015), payments from employers that fund the purchase of health insurance for retirees are considered taxable (Meacham 2014). If the Chamber had its way, the federal government would experience additional foregone revenue in relation to retirees' private health benefits. The preferential tax treatment that employers already enjoy for providing their workers' insurance is already the largest tax break under the federal tax code.

The Chamber staunchly opposes Medicare for All. As part of this campaign, it commissioned the firm Morning Consult to field a public opinion poll in December 2018 to illustrate how most Americans would rather stabilize the existing Medicare program than build a large, new government program. One of the key findings was that once respondents (2,000 registered voters) had heard a series of arguments designed to dissuade them from Medicare for All (there were no arguments offered in favor of Medicare for All as part of the survey), the percentages of supporters dropped by approximately one-half. Clearly, the project was designed to test weaknesses in the public's thinking about Medicare for All. Indicative of this strategy, the Chamber's CEO Thomas Donohue proclaimed in his State of American Business speech in January 2019 that "government-run, single-payer health care . . . doesn't work" and that the Chamber would "use all of our resources to combat it" (Luhby 2019). Based on what we see among several other pro-market groups profiled here, the Chamber will not be alone in this pursuit.

Sources

Abelson, Reed. 2019. "Hospitals Stand to Lose Millions under 'Medicare for All,'" *The New York Times* (September 23).

Alpern, Jonathan, William Stauffer, and Aaron Kesselheim. 2014. "High-Cost Generic Drugs—Implications for

Patients and Policy Makers." *New England Journal of Medicine* 371: 1,859–62.

American Hospital Association. 2019. "Underpayment by Medicare and Medicaid Fact Sheet" (January).

American Medical Association. 2018. "AMA Presents Government Service Award to Kaiser Family Foundation," press release (February 14).

American Medical Association. 2019. "Taking Steps Forward to Cover the Uninsured: Helping Low- and Moderate-Income Individuals Get Covered," policy document at AMA website.

America's Health Insurance Plans. 2019a. Amicus curiae brief filed with the U.S. Court of Appeals for the 5th Circuit (April 1).

America's Health Insurance Plans. 2019b. "Medicare for All & Health Care's Path Forward: AHIP CEO," press release (September 12).

Angell, Marcia. 2015. "Why Do Drug Companies Charge So Much? Because They Can," *The Washington Post* (September 25).

Antos, Joseph, and James Capretta. 2019. "Assessing the Effects of a Rebate Rollback on Drug Prices and Spending," *Health Affairs Blog* (March 11).

Armstrong, Drew, and John Tozzi. 2019. "Biggest U.S. Health Insurer Wades Right into 'Medicare for All' Fight," *Bloomberg News* (April 16).

Axos. 2018. "PhRMA Spends Money on Conservative Think Tanks, Political Groups, and Patient Advocates" (November 20).

Bach, Peter. 2016. "How the U.S. Could Cure Drug Price Insanity," *Forbes* (September 17).

Business Wire. 2019. "UnitedHealth Group Reports 2018 Results Highlighted by Continued Strong and Diversified Growth," press release (January 15).

Castillo, Bonnie. 2019. "Nurses across the U.S. Just Endorsed Bernie Sanders—Here's Why," *The Hill* (November 23).

Center for Responsive Politics. 2019. "Client Profile: American Medical Association." Available at www.crp.org.

Center for Responsive Politics. 2020. "Profile for 2018 Election Cycle, U.S. Chamber of Commerce." Available at www.crp.org.

Cunningham, Paige. 2015. "Meet the Group Blocking Obamacare's Medicaid Expansion," *The Washington Examiner* (April 8).

Darby, Luke. 2019. "Why Nurses Are Going Door-to-Door for Medicare for All," *GQ Magazine* (June 28).

Fuchs, Victor. 2018. "Is Single Payer the Answer for the U.S. Health Care System?" *Journal of the American Medical Association* 319 (1): 15–16.

Hancock, Jay. 2018. "Drug Trade Group Quietly Spends 'Dark Money' to Sway Public and Voters," *Kaiser Health News* (July 30).

Hertel-Fernandez, Alexander, Theda Skocpol, and Jason Sclar. 2018. "When Political Mega-Donors Join Forces: How the Koch Network and the Democracy Alliance Influence Organized U.S. Politics on the Right and Left." *Studies in American Political Development* 32 (October): 127–65.

Japsen, Bruce. 2019a. "Doctors Support 'Medicare for Some,'" *Forbes* (March 3).

Japsen, Bruce. 2019b. "Trump's Aborted Drug Price Rule Spares 'Middlemen' and the Drug Industry," *Forbes* (July 11).

Kacik, Alex. 2017. "American Hospital Association Restructures to Focus on Advocacy," *Modern Health Care* (December 8).

Kaiser Family Foundation. 2016. "10 Essential Facts about Medicare and Prescription Drug Spending" (January 29).

Kliff, Sarah. 2016. "What Bernie Sanders Can Learn about Single-Payer from His Home State of Vermont," *Vox News* (January 20).

Lexology. 2019. "CMS Issues Controversial Health Care Pricing and Insurance Coverage Transparency Rules" (November 20).

Liss, Samantha. 2018. "CEO Matt Lyles on Why AHIP Will Probably Have to Change Its Name," *Healthcaredive.com* (October 23).

Livingston, Shelby. 2018. "Insurers Profit from Medicare Advantage's Incentive to Add Coding that Boosts Reimbursement," *Modern Healthcare* (September 1).

Luhby, Tami. 2019. "Opponents Line Up to Quash Medicare for All," Cable News Network, February 25.

Luthi, Susannah. 2019. "AMA Exits Partnership Fighting Medicare for All, Public Options," *Modern Healthcare* (August 15).

Meacham, Jane. 2014. "Accident, Health Premiums Paid by Retirement Plans Become Taxable in 2015," report for HR Advisor (May 9).

Meyer, Harris. 2019. "Seema Verma's Bold Initiatives Land Her in No. 1 Most Influential Spot," Modern Healthcare (December 6).

Morse, Susan. 2018. "Humana Splits from AHIP, Third Large Insurer in Three Years to Leave," *Health Care Financial News* (January 10).

National Law Review. 2020. "Federal District Court Upholds Hospital Price Transparency Rule; Implementation and Compliance Questions Remain" (June 26).

National Nurses United. 2019. "Largest U.S. Nurses' Union Champions New Medicare for All House Bill," press release (February 26).

Oliver, Thomas, Philip Lee, and Helene Lipton. 2004. "A Political History of Medicare and Prescription Drug Coverage." *The Milbank Quarterly* 82 (2): 283–354.

Pear, Robert. 2019. "Health Care and Insurance Industries Mobilize to Kill 'Medicare for All,' " *The New York Times* (February 23).

Physicians for a National Health Program. 2019. "Doctors rally for Medicare for All, Demand Rep. Dwight Evans Co-Sponsor Single-Payer Legislation," press release (November 2).

Pollack, Andrew. 2015. "Drug Companies Increasingly Pushed to Explain High Prices," *The New York Times* (July 23).

Pollack, Rick. 2019. "Perspective: Is 'Medicare for All' the Right Answer?" American Hospital Association (February 22).

Porter, Steven. 2019. "R.I.P. Rebate Rule: Centerpiece Plucked from Trump's Drug Pricing Blueprint," *HealthLeaders Analysis* (July 11).

Potter, Wendell, and Nick Penniman. 2016. *Nation on the Take: How Big Money Corrupts Our Democracy and What We Can Do about It.* New York: Bloomsbury Press.

Roarty, Alex. 2014. "A Conservative Juggernaut's Long Game," *The Atlantic* (June 16).

Roy, Avik. 2019. "Trump's New Pharmacy Benefit Manager Rebate Rule Will Reshape Prescription Drug Prices," *Forbes* (February 2).

Shaw, Greg M. 2017. *The Dysfunctional Politics of the Affordable Care Act.* Santa Barbara, CA: Praeger.

Shih, Chuck, Jordan Schwartz, and Allan Coukell. 2016. "How Would Government Negotiation of Medicare Part D Drug Prices Work?" *Health Affairs Blog* (February 1).

Stein, Jeff. 2019. "'We've Done a Lot More Than You Would Think': How the Health-Insurance Industry Is Working to Pull Democrats Away from Medicare-for-All," *The Washington Post* (April 12).

Stolberg, Sheryl. 2013. "States Are Focus of Effort to Foil Health Care Law," *The New York Times* (October 18).

198   Medicare and Medicaid

Sullivan, Peter. 2019. "American Medical Association Leaves Coalition Fighting 'Medicare for All,'" *The Hill* (August 15).

UnitedHealth Group PAC. 2019. "U.S. Political Contributions & Related Activity."

U.S. Chamber of Commerce. 2001. "U.S. Chamber Affiliate Launches Ad Campaign to Oppose Kennedy-McCain Legislation," press release (June 14).

Vozzella, Laura. 2019. "Republicans Who Helped Expand Medicaid in Virginia Mostly Escape Primary Challenges," *The Washington Post* (June 14).

Ward, Nicholas. 2019. "UnitedHealth: Political Fears Are Creating Attractive Value," Thestreet.com (October 4).

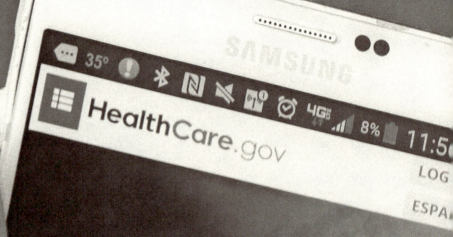

SAMSUNG

35° 📶 4G 8% 11:5
HealthCare.gov
LOG
ESPA

Open Enrollment for 2016 is here

First time applying on HealthCare.gov?

TAKE THE FIRST STEP TO APPLY

Have a 2015 Marketplace plan?

LOG IN TO KEEP/CHANGE

5 Data and Documents

This chapter includes a collection of graphs and documents that highlight some of the key accomplishments of Medicare and Medicaid over the past half century. Speeches by notable politicians also highlight their aspirations and hesitations about these programs. The language Lyndon Johnson used in 1965 when signing Medicare and Medicaid into law spoke of the long struggle for health care security and praised the then-former President Harry Truman for his part in that effort. President Obama's comments upon signing the Affordable Care Act into law in 2010 also referenced what he and his allies saw as the great accomplishment of extending health insurance to millions more Americans. However, other commentators were not so sanguine. U.S. Senator Lamar Alexander of Tennessee in 2009 spoke from the floor of the Senate to register his objection to the proposed expansion of Medicaid under the ACA. Building on this perspective, Chief Justice John Roberts codified his disapproval in his 2012 majority opinion finding that to make the Medicaid expansion obligatory for states violated the Constitution. For their part, the Medicare Trustees—the official auditors of the program—wrote in their 2019 report to Congress of the coming failure of the Medicare's Hospital Insurance Trust Fund, meaning that the program would not be able to meets its full obligations unless Congress addresses the funding mechanisms. Beyond these excerpted documents, this

---

Millions of Americans have used the healthcare.gov website to sign up for health insurance since 2014. (Tracy King/Dreamstime.com)

chapter also includes graphs showing program usage and expenditure trends across time, the percent of Americans still lacking health insurance, and other vital data on these programs.

DATA

Figure 5.1. Medicaid Enrollment by Year (1968–2018)

Because of the generous federal funding that Medicaid offers, states were quick to adopt it, bringing the national enrollment up to approximately 20 million by the mid-1970s. However, because the initial design was one that targeted assistance to narrow categories—children, single parents, senior citizens, and the disabled—the roles essentially stagnated until Congress gradually expanded eligibility through the 1980s into the 1990s. This series of steps had the effect of severing the relationship between welfare and Medicaid, reflected in the enrollment numbers in figure 5.1.

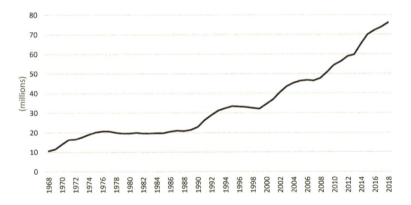

Figure 5.1.
Source: Centers for Medicare and Medicaid Services

Figure 5.2. Medicaid Spending by Year (1968–2018)

In response to the growing Medicaid rolls, especially beginning in the 1990s, the overall cost of the program grew significantly from that point forward. The expansion of eligibility, combined with the medical inflation rate (steeper since the early 1980s than it was before), the cost of the program has come to consume a much larger portion of both federal and state budgets than was the case during

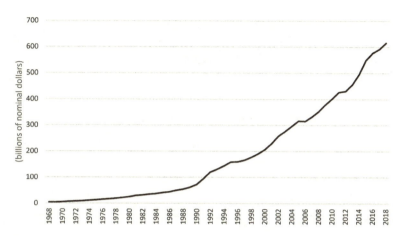

Figure 5.2.
Source: Centers for Medicare and Medicaid Services

the first couple of decades of the program. The expenditure trend, in nominal dollars, appears in figure 5.2.

Figure 5.3. Medicaid Enrollment by Age Group as a Percentage of Total (2017)

Although Medicaid spends most of its funds on long-term care for the chronically ill and the elderly, the large majority of its beneficiaries are low-income children and their parents. This pattern

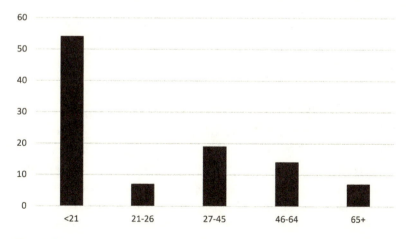

Figure 5.3.
Source: Centers for Medicare and Medicaid Services

has held for the past several decades. This duality reinforces the program's importance in contemporary health care financing. Two different demographic groups are key beneficiaries, but they rely on the program for very different types of services.

Figure 5.4. Medicare Enrollment by Year (1968–2018)

As with Medicaid, the number of Americans who benefit from Medicare has risen dramatically over time. This is attributable to an aging population, bearing in mind that the eligibility age of 65 has remained constant since the program's inception. As of 2018, some 60 million Americans, just over 18 percent of the nation's population, were enrolled in Medicare.

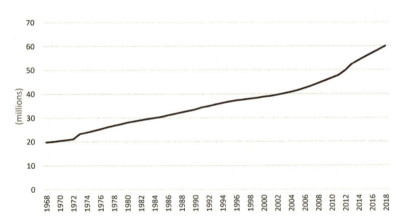

Figure 5.4.
Source: Medicare Trustees Reports

Figure 5.5. Medicare Spending by Year (1968–2018)

Like the steep rise in Medicaid spending shown in figure 5.2, Medicare expenditures have also tracked upward at an accelerating pace, particularly since the late 1980s. The two primary factors in this rise have been the aging of the baby boomers, with more of them now enrolled, and rising per capita expenditures under the program. The rise in per capita spending is attributable to

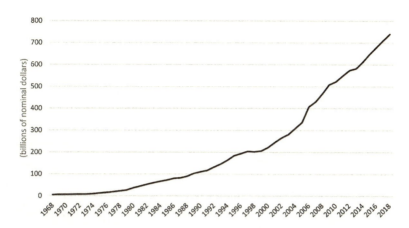

Figure 5.5.

Source: Medicare Trustees Reports, and Historical Tables of the Budget of the United States

aging. Older people tend to consume more medical services than do younger people, and this is especially true during the last couple of years of life. Further, advancing medical technology offers more expensive services.

Figure 5.6. Medicare Advantage Enrollment (1999–2019)

In the late 1990s, Congress offered the option of managed care to Medicare enrollees. This was attractive for seniors who wanted to avoid expensive co-payments. In exchange, these persons are typically limited in the range of providers they may access. In addition to pleasing seniors, policy makers also hoped that applying managed care models to Medicare would limit the program's expenditures. This latter expectation has not been realized (see Chapter 2 for discussion). However, what is now called Medicare Advantage has grown in popularity, as figure 5.6 illustrates. As of 2019, fully over 22 million Medicare beneficiaries elected this coverage model, and this number is expected to continue to rise. That the average Medicare Advantage enrollee costs the program a few percentage

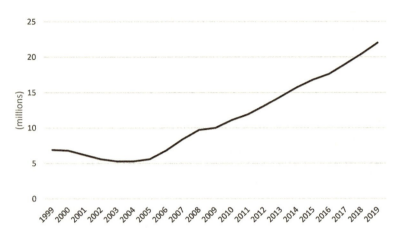

Figure 5.6.
Source: Centers for Medicare and Medicaid Services

points more than does the average senior enrolled in traditional Medicare is not only a vexing problem for policy makers but also one that defies current efforts to remedy.

Figure 5.7. The Uninsured Rate (1997–2018)

The efforts undertaken by the Affordable Care Act of 2010 to make health insurance available to more people have been quite successful, as figure 5.7 shows. Since 2010, approximately 20 million more Americans have gained coverage, mainly through the Medicaid expansion, but also through the online marketplaces operated by states and the federal government. Also visible in this graph is the rise in the number of uninsured people through the first decade of the 21st century, a trend that helped put health care reform on the agenda around the time of Barack Obama's election to the presidency. The United States Census Bureau tracks the percentage of those without health insurance for an entire year, and their American Community Survey is generally accepted as the definitive count. In 2018, this survey found that 8.5 percent Americans went the entire year without coverage. A slightly higher percentage of the population went at least part of each year without health insurance. These latter figures are not shown here. Such estimates

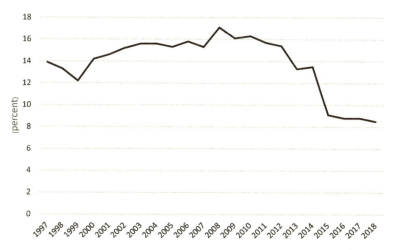

Figure 5.7.
Source: U.S. Census Bureau, American Community Survey, various years

are collected, for example, by the Gallup Organization a few times each year in national surveys.

According to the Census Bureau, in 2018 most uninsured people—72 percent—lived in low-income families with at least one full-time worker. The vast majority—86 percent—of America's uninsured are non-elderly adults. The uninsured rate that year among children was just 5 percent. This low rate among children is largely due to the broad coverage offered by the Children's Health Insurance Program, illustrated in figure 5.8 below.

Figure 5.8. Enrollment in the Children's Health Insurance Program (1998–2018)

When Congress created the CHIP program as part of the Balanced Budget Act of 1997, the Clinton Administration and legislators envisioned this as a modest add-on to Medicaid. States would be allowed to enroll children in families with income above their respective states' eligibility guidelines, even though their parents would not be eligible for this expanded assistance. Helping children is usually politically easier than helping working-age

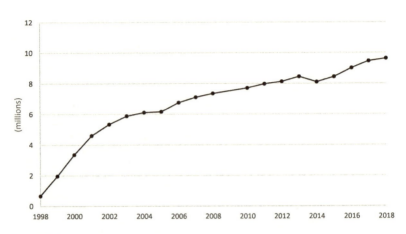

Figure 5.8.
Source: Kaiser Family Foundation, "Total Number of Children Ever Enrolled in CHIP Annually," based on data from the Centers for Medicare and Medicaid Services

adults. As their option, states quickly adopted the program, and the more generous ones added tens of thousands of children above and beyond those who would normally receive Medicaid. Upon its 10-year reauthorization in 2007, Democrats attempted to expand the program, allowing in children from families with incomes approaching middle-class. President George W. Bush vetoed this attempt, though President Obama approved an expansion early in his first term.

DOCUMENTS

President Lyndon Johnson's Remarks upon Signing Medicare and Medicaid into Law (1965)

President Johnson signed Medicare and Medicaid into law at the Harry Truman Library in Independence, Missouri, on July 30, 1965. With Truman sitting at his side, Johnson praised the former president's efforts to enact a broad health program and commented on the good that these new programs would do for the American people. He briefly explained some of the benefits these

*programs deliver for their beneficiaries with a particular focus on
low-income individuals.*

. . . The people of the United States love and voted for Harry
Truman, not because he gave them hell—but because he gave
them hope. I believe today that all America shares my joy that
he is present now when the hope that he offered becomes a
reality for millions of our fellow citizens. I am so proud that
this has come to pass in the Johnson administration. But it
was really Harry Truman of Missouri who planted the seeds
of compassion and duty, which have today flowered into care
for the sick, and serenity for the fearful. Many men can make
many proposals. . . . But few have the piercing and humane
eye, which can see beyond the words to the people that they
touch. Few can see past the speeches and the political battles
to the doctor over there that is tending the infirm, and to the
hospital that is receiving those in anguish, or feel in their heart
painful wrath at the injustice which denies the miracle of healing to the old and to the poor. And fewer still have the courage
to stake reputation, and position, and the effort of a lifetime
upon such a cause when there are so few that share it. But it
is just such men who illuminate the life and the history of a
nation.

And so, President Harry Truman, it is in tribute not to you,
but to the America that you represent, that we have come here
to pay our love and our respects to you today. . . . It was
a generation ago that Harry Truman said, and I quote him:
"Millions of our citizens do not now have a full measure of
opportunity to achieve and to enjoy good health. Millions
do not now have protection or security against the economic
effects of sickness. And the time has now arrived for action
to help them attain that opportunity and to help them get
that protection." Well, today, Mr. President, and my fellow
Americans, we are taking such action—20 years later. There
are more than 18 million Americans over the age of 65. Most
of them have low incomes. Most of them are threatened by

illness and medical expenses that they cannot afford. And through this new law, Mr. President, every citizen will be able, in his productive years when he is earning, to insure himself against the ravages of illness in his old age. This insurance will help pay for care in hospitals, in skilled nursing homes, or in the home. And under a separate plan it will help meet the fees of the doctors.

Now here is how the plan will affect you. During your working years, the people of America . . . will contribute through the Social Security program a small amount each payday for hospital insurance protection. For example, the average worker in 1966 will contribute about $1.50 per month. The employer will contribute a similar amount. And this will provide the funds to pay up to 90 days of hospital care for each illness, plus diagnostic care, and up to 100 home health visits after you are 65. And beginning in 1967, you will also be covered for up to 100 days of care in a skilled nursing home after a period of hospital care. And under a separate plan, when you are 65 . . . you may be covered for medical and surgical fees whether you are in or out of the hospital. You will pay $3 per month after you are 65 and your government will contribute an equal amount. The benefits under the law are as varied and broad as the marvelous modern medicine itself. . . . No longer will older Americans be denied the healing miracle of modern medicine. No longer will illness crush and destroy the savings that they have so carefully put away over a lifetime so that they might enjoy dignity in their later years. No longer will young families see their own incomes, and their own hopes, eaten away simply because they are carrying out their deep moral obligations to their parents, and to their uncles, and their aunts. And no longer will this nation refuse the hand of justice to those who have given a lifetime of service and wisdom and labor to the progress of this progressive country. And this bill . . . will increase Social Security benefits for all of our older Americans. It will improve a wide range of health and medical services for Americans of all ages.

In 1935 when the man that both of us loved so much, Franklin Delano Roosevelt, signed the Social Security Act, he said it was, and I quote him, "a cornerstone in a structure which is being built but it is by no means complete." Well, perhaps no single act in the entire administration of the beloved Franklin D. Roosevelt really did more to win him the illustrious place in history that he has, as did the laying of that cornerstone. But it all started really with the man from Independence. And so, as it is fitting that we should, we have come back here to his home to complete what he began. President Harry Truman . . . made many decisions of great moment; although he always made them frankly and with a courage and a clarity that few men have ever shared . . .

. . . There is another tradition that we share today. It calls upon us never to be indifferent toward despair. It commands us never to turn away from helplessness. It directs us never to ignore or to spurn those who suffer untended in a land that is bursting with abundance . . . The highest traditions of the medical profession are really directed to the ends that we are trying to serve. And it was only yesterday, at the request of some of my friends, I met with the leaders of the American Medical Association to seek their assistance in advancing the cause of one of the greatest professions of all—the medical profession—in helping us to maintain and to improve the health of all Americans. And this is not just our tradition—or the tradition of the Democratic Party—or even the tradition of the Nation. It is as old as the day it was first commanded: "Thou shalt open thine hand wide unto thy brother, to thy poor, to thy needy, in thy land." And just think, Mr. President, because of this document—and the long years of struggle which so many have put into creating it—in this town, and a thousand other towns like it, there are men and women in pain who will now find ease. There are those, alone in suffering who will now hear the sound of some approaching footsteps coming to help. There are those fearing the terrible darkness of despairing poverty—despite their long years of labor and expectation—who will now look up to see the light of hope and realization. There just can be no satisfaction, nor any act of leadership, that gives greater satisfaction than this. And perhaps you alone, President Truman, perhaps you alone can fully know just how grateful I am for this day."

Source: *Public Papers of the Presidents of the United States.* Lyndon B. Johnson: 1965, Book 2. Washington, D.C.: Government Printing Office, 1966, 811–814.

President Barack Obama's Remarks upon Signing the Patient Protection and Affordable Care Act into Law (2010)

President Obama signed the ACA into law on March 23, 2010, at the White House. Surrounded by congressional leaders and select citizens who would benefit from the ACA's expansion of coverage, Obama talked about how this represented a bold step forward, which had required a great deal of courage from advocates over many years. He spoke about how the new law would help a broad swath of Americans and how its consumer protections would assist people who had struggled to secure insurance coverage in the private market. This was particularly relevant since much of the coverage expansion under the ACA would later involve the combination of government subsidies and private insurers.

Today, after almost a century of trying, today, after over a year of debate, today, after all the votes have been tallied, health insurance reform becomes law in the United States of America—today. It is fitting that Congress passed this historic legislation this week. For as we mark the turning of spring, we also mark a new season in America. In a few moments, when I sign this bill, all of the overheated rhetoric over reform will finally confront the reality of reform . . . The bill I'm signing will set in motion reforms that generations of Americans have fought for and marched for and hungered to see. It will take four years to implement fully many of these reforms, because we need to implement them responsibly. We need to get this right. But a host of desperately needed reforms will take effect right away. This year, we'll start offering tax credits to about four million small business men and women to help them cover the cost of insurance for their employees. That happens this year. This year, tens of thousands of uninsured Americans with preexisting conditions, the parents of children who have a preexisting condition, will finally be able to purchase the coverage they need. That happens this year. This year, insurance companies will no longer be able to drop people's coverage when they get sick. They won't be able to place lifetime limits or restrictive annual limits on the amount of care they can receive. This year, all new insurance plans will be required to offer free preventive care. And this year, young adults will be able to stay on their parents' policies until they're 26 years old. That happens this year. And this year, seniors who fall in the coverage gap known as the doughnut hole will start getting some help. They'll receive $250 to help pay for prescriptions, and that will, over time, fill in the doughnut hole. And I want seniors to know, despite what some have said, these reforms will not cut your guaranteed benefits. In fact, under this law, Americans on Medicare will receive free preventive care without co-payments or deductibles. That begins this year. Once this reform is implemented, health insurance exchanges will be created, a competitive marketplace where uninsured people and small businesses will finally be able to purchase affordable, quality insurance. They will be able to be part of a big pool and get the same good deal that members of Congress get. That's what's going to happen under this reform. And when this exchange is up and running millions of people will get tax breaks to help them afford coverage, which represents the largest middle-class tax cut for health care in history. That's what this reform is about.

This legislation will also lower costs for families and for businesses and for the Federal Government, reducing our deficit by over $1 trillion in the next two decades. It is paid for, it is fiscally responsible, and it will help lift a decades-long drag on our economy. That's part of what all of you together worked on and made happen. That our generation is able to succeed in passing this reform is a testament to the persistence and the character of the American people, who championed this cause, who mobilized, who organized, who believed that people who love this country can change it. It's also a testament to the historic leadership and uncommon courage of the men and women of the United States Congress, who've taken their lumps during this difficult debate. But we're still standing. You know, there are few tougher jobs in politics or government than leading one of our legislative chambers . . . It isn't always tidy; it is almost never easy. But perhaps the greatest and most difficult challenge is to cobble together out of those differences the sense of common interest and common purpose that's required to advance the dreams of all people, especially in a country as large and diverse as ours . . .

Today I'm signing this reform bill into law on behalf of my mother, who argued with insurance companies even as she battled cancer in her final days. I'm signing it for Ryan Smith, who's here today. He runs a small business with five employees. He's trying to do the right thing, paying half the cost of coverage for his workers. This bill will help him afford that coverage . . . I'm signing this bill for all the leaders who took up this cause through the generations, from Teddy Roosevelt to Franklin Roosevelt, from Harry Truman to Lyndon Johnson, from Bill and Hillary Clinton . . . Our presence here today is remarkable and improbable . . . It's easy to succumb to the sense of cynicism about what's possible in this country. But today we are affirming that essential truth, a truth every generation is called to rediscover for itself, that we are not a nation that scales back its aspirations. We are not a nation that falls prey to doubt or mistrust. We don't fall prey to fear. We are not a nation that does what's easy. That's not who we are. That's not how we got here. We are a nation that faces its challenges and accepts its responsibilities. We are a nation that does what is hard, what is necessary, what is right. Here in this country, we shape our own destiny. That is what we do. That is who we are. That is what makes us the United States of America. And we have now just enshrined, as soon as I sign this bill, the core principle that everybody should have some basic security when it comes to their health care. And it is an extraordinary achievement that has happened because of all of you and all the advocates all across the country. So thank you. Thank you. God bless you, and may God bless the United States of America.

Source: *Public Papers of the Presidents of the United States. Barack Obama: 2010, Book 1. Washington, D.C.: Government Printing Office, 2011, 400–402.*

U.S. Senator Lamar Alexander on the Proposed Expansion of Medicaid (2009)

Senator Alexander, a Republican and former governor of Tennessee, spoke on the floor of the U.S. Senate on October 26, 2009, about his opposition to the planned expansion of Medicaid, citing what he said would be an unbearable financial burden on state treasuries. He spoke for many when he addressed this issue, as numerous state officials expressed deep concern about what would become the ACA's financial impact on their budgets. Senator Alexander expressed his skepticism about the existing Medicaid program, his frustration with the expansion of the State Children's Health Insurance Program—initially passed in 1997 and expanded in 2009—and reiterated his belief that if members of Congress want to extent medical assistance to more Americans they should be prepared to pay for it and to not pass these expenses on to the states. Senator Alexander would later find an ally in Chief Justice John Roberts in the NFIB v. Sebelius decision, excerpted below, on this matter.

Mr. President, . . . [this] provides a good opportunity to talk about what we mean by a public option in health care, or a government-run health care plan, putting government in the health care business, and how it already works, and how it might work if States were allowed to opt out. The reason it is easy to talk about this is . . . we already have in existence in the United States today a public option health insurance program which States may opt out of. It is called Medicaid. Medicaid is the largest government-run program we have in health care—even larger than Medicare. Medicare, for older people, has about 40 million persons who depend on it. Medicaid, which sometimes offers confusion, is a different program. It is a program for low-income Americans. It started out for women and children, but it gradually expanded, and today it has nearly 60 million Americans who depend on it.

The [proposed] health care legislation . . . and the bills in the House of Representatives—all those pieces of legislation would expand the Medicaid Program . . . and send part of the bill for that expansion to the States. So let's talk about that a little bit, particularly if it is true that the majority leader is about to propose that we have yet another government-run insurance program, giving the States the right to opt out, which sounds pretty good. Let's see how this one works that we already have, especially since the health reform bill that is headed our way would expand Medicaid, and according to the Congressional Budget Office, cost States an additional $33 billion in State dollars and add 14 million people to Medicaid. I guess the first thing to know about a government-run health insurance program which States can opt out of is that they can't. I mean, in the real world, they can't. Not one has. Every State in America has Medicaid. The Federal Government pays roughly 60 percent of it; State taxpayers pay the rest. Most of the rules are written in Washington. States can ask for exemptions from the rules, but it is a long and burdensome process. It is not realistic to say the States can opt out of the Medicaid Program for low-income Americans. I suppose it might not be realistic, therefore, to say the States would be able to opt out of a new government-run program—a government-run, public-option program—hat may be suggested by the majority leader.

. . . I think we would be wise to pay attention to the fact that in the current government-run program we have today, no State finds it realistic to opt out. Expanding Medicaid, which is what the health reform bill coming toward us on the floor proposes to do, is not just an expensive item for the Federal Government and for States, it is a terrible vehicle for health care reform. The current Governor of Tennessee—Governor Bredesen—a Democrat—has said putting more low-income Americans into Medicaid is not health care reform. Why would he say that? Because it makes it worse for those Americans as they seek to get access to care from doctors and hospitals and as they seek to get good, quality care. Plus, the program is riddled with so much fraud and abuse that, according to the Congressional Budget Office, $1 out of every $10 is stolen or wasted. Most Governors who have struggled with Medicaid—and I am one of them—agree that its expansion is a bad idea. They unanimously have said to us in Congress that if you in Washington want to expand Medicaid, then you in Washington need to pay for Medicaid. That is the theory of no more unfunded mandates that every Governor whom I know about has agreed with for years. In fact, there was nothing that used to make me angrier as a Governor than for a distinguished politician in Washington to stand, make a speech, come up with a good idea, hold a press conference declaring a problem solved, and then send the bill to the States. So what does the Governor and the legislature and the mayor and the city council have to do? They have to cut services, they have to raise taxes, they have to run up tuition, they have to cut out some classes because somebody in Washington thought it was a good idea to do this. Well, that is what we are proposing to do with Medicaid. We are saying to the States: We have a great idea. We want to expand Medicaid by dumping another 14 million low-income Americans into this program, but congratulations, we are going to send you the bill to help pay for it . . .

[The previous Children's Health Insurance bill] unrealistically lifted the level of Medicaid spending in Tennessee and every other State, forcing an expansion of that program, which I will go on to show in a minute is nearly cruel to the people who are dumped into the program because doctors and hospitals will not serve them. So I was glad to vote against that program. I was sorry it passed because it borrowed money we don't have to spend on programs that didn't create jobs, and it artificially lifted and expanded Medicaid, which is already bankrupting the States.

Medicaid expansion is not real health care reform. One reason is because 40 percent—according to a 2002 Medicare Payment Advisory Committee survey—of the physicians restrict access for Medicaid patients; meaning they will not take new Medicaid patients because reimbursement rates are so low. Only about half of U.S. physicians accept new Medicaid patients compared with more than 70 percent who accept new Medicare—those are the seniors—patients. According to a 2002 study in the *Journal of American Academy of Pediatrics*, the national rate for pediatricians who accept all Medicaid patients was 55 percent. In Tennessee, it was lower than that. Why is that? It is because reimbursement rates are so low. Today, doctors who see patients who are on Medicare get paid about 80 percent of what private insurers pay. Doctors who see patients who are on Medicaid get paid about 61 or 62 percent of what private insurers pay. For doctors who see children, it is sometimes lower than that. So doctors don't see those patients. What is going to happen if we dump 14 more million low-income Americans into a system such as that? Those patients—especially those children—are going to have a harder time finding doctors and hospitals to taking care of them. It would be akin to giving somebody a ticket and a pat on the back to a bus line that only operated 50 percent of the time. Further, the quality of care for Medicaid patients is significantly lower than those with private insurance and even those with no insurance. According to a survey by the National Hospital Ambulatory Medical Care, Medicaid patients visit the emergency room at nearly twice the rate of uninsured patients. A 2007 study by the Journal of the American Medical Association found that patients enrolled in Medicaid were less likely to achieve good blood pressure control, receive breast cancer screening, have timely prenatal care than similar parents in private plans, and they had lower survival rates. I mentioned this a little earlier. According to the Government Accountability Office, Medicaid—the program we are seeking to expand, the government-run insurance program that sounds so good, the so-called largest public option plan we have to date, the plan where about half the doctors will not take new patients who are on the program—had $32.7 billion in improper payments in 2007 alone; 10 percent of the program's total spending is wasted. So as we consider a so-called public option, I hope we will look at the public option we already have—called Medicaid—one which already has an opt-out provision for States, one which already has 60 million low-income Americans in it, one into which we plan to put 14 million more Americans, so that 50 percent of the doctors will say to new patients: I can't see you because the reimbursement rates are so low. Medicaid is the public option we have right now. States could opt out of it, but quality is low, fraud is high, costs are up, and Governors of States on both sides of the aisle are saying: We are headed toward bankruptcy at the present rate. If you are sending us more bills, if you want to expand it, pay for it. And doctors are turning away patients. The American people deserve better than that . . .

Source: *Congressional Record.* Senate, Vol 155, Pt 19. October 26, 2009. Washington, D.C.: Government Printing Office, 25631–25633.

U.S. Supreme Court Ruling in *National Federation of Independent Businesses, et al. v. Kathleen Sebelius, Secretary of Health and Human Services, et al.* (2012)

On June 28, 2012, the Supreme Court ruled on two challenges to the Affordable Care Act. The first had to do with whether Congress has the constitutional authority to impose a fine on individuals who lack health insurance. The Court ruled that it did, under the power to tax found in Article I Section 8 of the Constitution. The second question was whether Congress could withhold all Medicaid funding from those states that declined to expand their Medicaid programs, as originally prescribed in the ACA. It ruled that such a sanction was not in line with contemporary understandings of American federalism, specifically that it represented federal coercion in an area that ought to remain the purview of the states.

Chief Justice Roberts announced the judgment of the Court . . . Today we resolve constitutional challenges to two provisions of the Patient Protection and Affordable Care Act of 2010: the individual mandate, which requires individuals to purchase a health insurance policy providing a minimum level of coverage; and the Medicaid expansion, which gives funds to the States on the condition that they provide specified health care to all citizens whose income falls below a certain threshold. We do not consider whether the Act embodies sound policies. That judgment is entrusted to the Nation's elected leaders. We ask only whether Congress has the power under the Constitution to enact the challenged provisions.

In our federal system, the National Government possesses only limited powers; the States and the people retain the remainder. Nearly two centuries ago, Chief Justice Marshall observed that "the question respecting the extent of the powers actually granted" to the Federal Government "is perpetually arising, and will probably continue to arise, as long as our system shall exist" (*McCulloch v. Maryland*, 1819). In this case we must again determine whether the Constitution grants Congress powers it now asserts, but which many States and individuals believe it does not possess. Resolving this controversy requires us to examine both the limits of the Government's power, and our own limited role in policing those boundaries.

The Federal Government "is acknowledged by all to be one of enumerated powers." That is, rather than granting general authority to perform all the conceivable functions of government, the Constitution lists, or enumerates, the Federal

Government's powers . . . The Constitution's express conferral of some powers makes clear that it does not grant others. And the Federal Government can exercise only the powers granted to it . . .

. . . This case concerns two powers that the Constitution does grant the Federal Government, but which must be read carefully to avoid creating a general federal authority akin to the police power. The Constitution authorizes Congress to "regulate Commerce with foreign Nations, and among the several States, and with the Indian Tribes." . . . Congress may also "lay and collect Taxes, Duties, Imposts and Excises, to pay the Debts and provide for the common Defence and general Welfare of the United States." . . . Put simply, Congress may tax and spend. This grant gives the Federal Government considerable influence even in areas where it cannot directly regulate. The Federal Government may enact a tax on an activity that it cannot authorize, forbid, or otherwise control . . . And in exercising its spending power, Congress may offer funds to the States, and may condition those offers on compliance with specified conditions . . .

. . . Our permissive reading of these powers is explained in part by a general reticence to invalidate the acts of the Nation's elected leaders. "Proper respect for a co-ordinate branch of the government" requires that we strike down an Act of Congress only if "the lack of constitutional authority to pass [the] act in question is clearly demonstrated." . . . Members of this Court are vested with the authority to interpret the law; we possess neither the expertise nor the prerogative to make policy judgments. Those decisions are entrusted to our Nation's elected leaders, who can be thrown out of office if the people disagree with them. It is not our job to protect the people from the consequences of their political choices. Our deference in matters of policy cannot, however, become abdication in matters of law. "The powers of the legislature are defined and limited; and that those limits may not be mistaken, or forgotten, the constitution is written." . . .

In 2010, Congress enacted the Patient Protection and Affordable Care Act . . . The Act aims to increase the number of Americans covered by health insurance and decrease the cost of health care. The Act's 10 titles stretch over 900 pages and contain hundreds of provisions. This case concerns constitutional challenges to two key provisions, commonly referred to as the individual mandate and the Medicaid expansion.

. . . The second provision of the Affordable Care Act directly challenged here is the Medicaid expansion. Enacted in 1965, Medicaid offers federal funding to States to assist pregnant women, children, needy families, the blind, the elderly, and the disabled in obtaining medical care . . . In order to receive that funding, States must comply with federal criteria governing matters such as who receives care and what services are provided at what cost. By 1982 every State had chosen to participate in Medicaid. Federal funds received through the Medicaid program have become a substantial part of state budgets . . .

The Affordable Care Act expands the scope of the Medicaid program and increases the number of individuals the States must cover. For example, the Act requires state programs to provide Medicaid coverage to adults with incomes up to 133 percent of the federal poverty level, whereas many States now cover adults with children only if their income is considerably lower, and do not cover childless adults at all . . . The Act increases federal funding to cover the States' costs in expanding Medicaid coverage, although States will bear a portion of the costs on their own . . . If a State does not comply with the Act's new coverage requirements, it may lose not only the federal funding for those requirements, but all of its federal Medicaid funds . . .

Along with their challenge to the individual mandate, the state plaintiffs in the Eleventh Circuit argued that the Medicaid expansion exceeds Congress's constitutional powers. The Court of Appeals unanimously held that the Medicaid expansion is a valid exercise of Congress's power under the

Spending Clause . . . And the court rejected the States' claim that the threatened loss of all federal Medicaid funding violates the Tenth Amendment by coercing them into complying with the Medicaid expansion . . .

. . . The States also contend that the Medicaid expansion exceeds Congress's authority under the Spending Clause. They claim that Congress is coercing the States to adopt the changes it wants by threatening to withhold all of a State's Medicaid grants, unless the State accepts the new expanded funding and complies with the conditions that come with it. This, they argue, violates the basic principle that the "Federal Government may not compel the States to enact or administer a federal regulatory program" . . . There is no doubt that the Act dramatically increases state obligations under Medicaid. The current Medicaid program requires States to cover only certain discrete categories of needy individuals—pregnant women, children, needy families, the blind, the elderly, and the disabled . . . There is no mandatory coverage for most childless adults, and the States typically do not offer any such coverage. The States also enjoy considerable flexibility with respect to the coverage levels for parents of needy families . . . On average States cover only those unemployed parents who make less than 37 percent of the federal poverty level, and only those employed parents who make less than 63 percent of the poverty line . . .

The Medicaid provisions of the Affordable Care Act, in contrast, require States to expand their Medicaid programs by 2014 to cover all individuals under the age of 65 with incomes below 133 percent of the federal poverty line . . . The Act also establishes a new "[e]ssential health benefits" package, which States must provide to all new Medicaid recipients—a level sufficient to satisfy a recipient's obligations under the individual mandate . . . The Affordable Care Act provides that the Federal Government will pay 100 percent of the costs of covering these newly eligible individuals through 2016 . . . In the following years, the federal payment level gradually decreases, to a minimum of 90 percent. In light of the expansion in coverage mandated by the Act, the Federal Government estimates that its Medicaid spending will increase by approximately $100 billion per year, nearly 40 percent above current levels . . .

. . . At the same time, our cases have recognized limits on Congress's power under the Spending Clause to secure state compliance with federal objectives. "We have repeatedly characterized . . . Spending Clause legislation as 'much in the nature of a contract.'" . . . The legitimacy of Congress's exercise of the spending power "thus rests on whether the State voluntarily and knowingly accepts the terms of the 'contract.'" . . . Respecting this limitation is critical to ensuring that Spending Clause legislation does not undermine the status of the States as independent sovereigns in our federal system. That system "rests on what might at first seem a counterintuitive insight, that 'freedom is enhanced by the creation of two governments, not one.'" . . . For this reason, "the Constitution has never been understood to confer upon Congress the ability to require the States to govern according to Congress' instructions." . . . Otherwise the two-government system established by the Framers would give way to a system that vests power in one central government, and individual liberty would suffer. That insight has led this Court to strike down federal legislation that commandeers a State's legislative or administrative apparatus for federal purposes . . . It has also led us to scrutinize Spending Clause legislation to ensure that Congress is not using financial inducements to exert a "power akin to undue influence." . . . Congress may use its spending power to create incentives for States to act in accordance with federal policies. But when "pressure turns into compulsion," the legislation runs contrary to our system of federalism. "[T]he Constitution simply does not give Congress the authority to require the States to regulate." . . . That is true whether Congress directly commands a State to regulate or indirectly coerces a State to adopt a federal regulatory system as its own.

Permitting the Federal Government to force the States to implement a federal program would threaten the political accountability key to our federal system. "[W]here the Federal Government directs the States to regulate, it may be state officials who will bear the brunt of public disapproval, while the federal officials who devised the regulatory program may remain insulated from the electoral ramifications of their decision." . . . Spending Clause programs do not pose this danger when a State has a legitimate choice whether to accept the federal conditions in exchange for federal funds. In such a situation, state officials can fairly be held politically accountable for choosing to accept or refuse the federal offer. But when the State has no choice, the Federal Government can achieve its objectives without accountability ... Indeed, this danger is heightened when Congress acts under the Spending Clause, because Congress can use that power to implement federal policy it could not impose directly under its enumerated powers.

. . . Instead of simply refusing to grant the new funds to States that will not accept the new conditions, Congress has also threatened [under the ACA] to withhold those States' existing Medicaid funds. The States claim that this threat serves no purpose other than to force unwilling States to sign up for the dramatic expansion in health care coverage effected by the Act.

Given the nature of the threat and the programs at issue here, we must agree. We have upheld Congress's authority to condition the receipt of funds on the States' complying with restrictions on the use of those funds, because that is the means by which Congress ensures that the funds are spent according to its view of the "general Welfare." Conditions that do not here govern the use of the funds, however, cannot be justified on that basis. When, for example, such conditions take the form of threats to terminate other significant independent grants, the conditions are properly viewed as a means of pressuring the States to accept policy changes.

. . . We accordingly asked whether "the financial inducement offered by Congress" was "so coercive as to pass the point at which 'pressure turns into compulsion.'" . . . In this case, the financial "inducement" Congress has chosen is much more than "relatively mild encouragement"—it is a gun to the head. Section 1396c of the Medicaid Act provides that if a State's Medicaid plan does not comply with the Act's requirements, the Secretary of Health and Human Services may declare that "further payments will not be made to the State." . . . A State that opts out of the Affordable Care Act's expansion in health care coverage thus stands to lose not merely "a relatively small percentage" of its existing Medicaid funding, but all of it . . . Medicaid spending accounts for over 20 percent of the average State's total budget, with federal funds covering 50 to 83 percent of those costs . . . The Federal Government estimates that it will pay out approximately $3.3 trillion between 2010 and 2019 in order to cover the costs of pre-expansion Medicaid . . . The Medicaid expansion, however, accomplishes a shift in kind, not merely degree ... Under the Affordable Care Act, Medicaid is transformed into a program to meet the health care needs of the entire nonelderly population with income below 133 percent of the poverty level. It is no longer a program to care for the neediest among us, but rather an element of a comprehensive national plan to provide universal health insurance coverage. . . . Indeed, the manner in which the expansion is structured indicates that while Congress may have styled the expansion a mere alteration of existing Medicaid, it recognized it was enlisting the States in a new health care program . . . Congress may not simply "conscript state [agencies] into the national bureaucratic army" . . . and that is what it is attempting to do with the Medicaid expansion.

. . . The Affordable Care Act is constitutional in part and unconstitutional in part. The individual mandate cannot be upheld as an exercise of Congress's power under the Commerce Clause. That Clause authorizes Congress to regulate interstate commerce, not to order individuals to engage in it. In this case, however, it is reasonable to construe what Congress has done as increasing taxes on those who have a certain amount of income, but choose to go without health insurance. Such legislation is within Congress's power to tax.

As for the Medicaid expansion, that portion of the Affordable Care Act violates the Constitution by threatening existing
Medicaid funding ... Congress may offer the States grants and
require the States to comply with accompanying conditions,
but the States must have a genuine choice whether to accept
the offer. The States are given no such choice in this case: They
must either accept a basic change in the nature of Medicaid, or
risk losing all Medicaid funding. The remedy for that constitutional violation is to preclude the Federal Government from
imposing such a sanction ... The Framers created a Federal
Government of limited powers, and assigned to this Court the
duty of enforcing those limits. The Court does so today. But
the Court does not express any opinion on the wisdom of the
Affordable Care Act. Under the Constitution, that judgment is
reserved to the people.

The judgment of the Court of Appeals for the Eleventh Circuit is affirmed in part and reversed in part. It is so ordered.

Source: *National Federation of Independent Business v. Sebelius,*
567 U.S. 519 (2012).

Report of the Boards of Trustees of the Federal Hospital Insurance and Federal Supplementary Medical Insurance Trust Funds (2019)

*Each spring, the Medicare Trustees issue a report to Congress and
the public with their audit of the program and projections for
future performance. Throughout recent years, the Trustees have
noted that the funding for the Supplemental Medical Insurance
Fund, which pays for Part B, is projected to be solvent for the next
75 years; the Trustees have warned of coming deficits in the Hospital Insurance Trust Fund, the fund that pays for Part A. This latter
fund is projected to be unable to meet its full obligations starting in 2026. Congress basically has two alternatives: reduce the
amounts paid to providers under Part A of Medicare or restructure
the revenue stream for this part of the program. The latter could be*

accomplished by a tax increase, or a decision to spend general revenue funds on Medicare, or a combination of both. In an effort to reduce entitlement program spending, the Trump Administration has proposed shaving hundreds of billions of dollars off Medicare spending over the coming decade, though Congress has not given this proposal serious attention.

. . . Projections of Medicare costs are highly uncertain, especially when looking out more than several decades. One reason for uncertainty is that scientific advances will make possible new interventions, procedures, and therapies. Some conditions that are untreatable today will be handled routinely in the future. Spurred by economic incentives, the institutions through which care is delivered will evolve, possibly becoming more efficient. While most health care technological advances to date have tended to increase expenditures, the health care landscape is shifting. No one knows whether future developments will, on balance, increase or decrease costs. Certain features of current law may result in some challenges for the Medicare program. Physician payment update amounts are specified for all years in the future, and these amounts do not vary based on underlying economic conditions, nor are they expected to keep pace with the average rate of physician cost increases. These rate updates could be an issue in years when levels of inflation are high and would be problematic when the cumulative gap between the price updates and physician costs becomes large . . .

Medicare beneficiaries would, under current law, fall over time compared to that received by those with private health insurance. Since 1960, U.S. national health expenditure (NHE) growth rates typically outpaced economic growth rates, though the magnitude of the differences has been declining. The Trustees have long assumed that this differential would continue to narrow over the long-term projection period and that the cost-reduction provisions of the Patient Protection and Affordable Care Act . . . and the Medicare Access and CHIP Reauthorization Act of 2015 (MACRA) would further decrease this gap.

Data and Documents 229

Since 2008, average annual NHE growth has been below historical averages, though it has generally continued to outpace average annual growth of the economy. There is some debate regarding whether this recent slower growth in national health expenditures reflects the impact of economic factors that are mostly cyclical in nature, such as modest income growth over the last decade, or factors that would lead to a permanently slower growth environment, such as structural changes to the health sector that could result in lower health care cost growth. The Trustees' outlook for long-range NHE growth is consistent with the trajectory observed over the past half century and has not been materially affected by this recent experience. Notwithstanding recent favorable developments, current-law projections indicate that Medicare still faces a substantial financial shortfall that will need to be addressed with further legislation. Such legislation should be enacted sooner rather than later to minimize the impact on beneficiaries, providers, and taxpayers . . .

The current-law expenditure projections reflect the physicians' payment levels expected under the MACRA payment rules and the ACA-mandated reductions in other Medicare payment rates, but not the payment reductions and/or delays that would result from the HI trust fund depletion. In the year of asset depletion, which is projected to be 2026 in this report, HI revenues are projected to cover 89 percent of program costs . . .

Medicare's costs under current law rise steadily from their current level of 3.7 percent of GDP in 2018 to 6.0 percent in 2043. Costs then continue to grow, but at a slower rate, until reaching 6.5 percent in 2093. . . . The estimated depletion date for the HI trust fund is 2026, the same as in last year's report. As in past years, the Trustees have determined that the fund is not adequately financed over the next 10 years. HI income is projected to be lower than last year's estimates due to lower payroll taxes and lower income from the taxation of Social Security benefits. HI expenditures are projected to be slightly higher than last year's estimates because of higher-than-projected 2018 spending and higher projected provider payment updates, factors that are mostly offset by the effect of lower assumed utilization of skilled nursing facility services. In 2018, HI expenditures exceeded income by $1.6 billion. The Trustees project deficits in all future years until the trust fund becomes depleted in 2026. The assets were $200.4 billion at the beginning of 2019, representing about 62 percent of expenditures during the year, which is below the Trustees' minimum recommended level of 100 percent. The HI trust fund has not met the Trustees' formal test of short-range financial adequacy since 2003. Growth in HI expenditures has averaged 3.0 percent annually over the last 5 years, compared with noninterest income growth of 4.4 percent. Over the next 5 years, projected annual growth rates for expenditures and noninterest income are 7.0 percent and 5.7 percent, respectively. The Supplemental Medical Insurance trust fund is expected to be adequately financed over the next 10 years and beyond because income from premiums and general revenue for Parts B and D are reset each year to cover expected costs and ensure a reserve for Part B contingencies. The monthly Part B premium for 2019 is $135.50. Part B and Part D costs have averaged annual growth rates of 6.6 percent and 6.3 percent, respectively, over the last 5 years, as compared to growth of 4.1 percent for GDP. Under current law, the Trustees project that cost growth over the next 5 years will average 8.3 percent for Part B and 7.3 percent for Part D, significantly faster than the projected average annual GDP growth rate of 4.7 percent over the period.

The Trustees are issuing a determination of projected excess general revenue Medicare funding in this report because the difference between Medicare's total outlays and its dedicated financing sources is projected to exceed 45 percent of outlays within 7 years. Since this determination was made last year as well, this year's determination triggers a Medicare funding warning, which (i) requires the President to submit to Congress proposed legislation to respond to the warning within 15 days after the submission of the Fiscal Year 2021 Budget and (ii) requires Congress to consider the legislation on an expedited basis. This is the third consecutive year that a determination of excess general revenue Medicare funding has been issued, and the second consecutive year that a Medicare funding warning has been issued.

. . . The long-range projections as a percent of GDP are somewhat higher than those projected last year due to faster projected spending growth for physician-administered drugs and slower assumed growth of economy-wide productivity. (Part B costs in 2093 would be 4.5 percent under the illustrative alternative scenario.) The Board estimates that Part D outlays will increase from 0.5 percent of GDP in 2018 to about 1.1 percent by 2093. These long-range outlay projections, as a percent of GDP, are slightly lower than those shown in last year's report. Transfers from the general fund finance about three-quarters of SMI costs and are central to the automatic financial balance of the fund's two accounts. Such transfers represent a large and growing requirement for the Federal budget. SMI general revenues equal 1.6 percent of GDP in 2018 and are projected to increase to an estimated 3.0 percent in 2093 . . .

Total Medicare expenditures were $741 billion in 2018. The Board projects that expenditures will increase in future years at a faster pace than either aggregate workers' earnings or the economy overall and that, as a percentage of GDP, they will increase from 3.7 percent in 2018 to 6.5 percent by 2093 (based on the Trustees' intermediate set of assumptions). If the relatively low price increases for physicians and other health services under Medicare are not sustained and do not take full effect in the long range as assumed in the illustrative alternative projection, then Medicare spending would instead represent roughly 9.0 percent of GDP in 2093.

Growth under any of these scenarios, if realized, would substantially increase the strain on the nation's workers, the economy, Medicare beneficiaries, and the Federal budget. The Trustees project that HI tax income and other dedicated revenues will fall short of HI expenditures in all future years. The HI trust fund does not meet either the Trustees' test of short-range financial adequacy or their test of long-range close actuarial balance. The Part B and Part D accounts in the SMI trust fund are expected to be adequately financed because income from premiums and general revenue are reset each year to cover expected costs. Such financing, however, would have to increase faster than the economy to cover expected expenditure growth.

The financial projections in this report indicate a need for substantial changes to address Medicare's financial challenges. The sooner solutions are enacted, the more flexible and gradual they can be. The early introduction of reforms increases the time available for affected individuals and organizations—including health care providers, beneficiaries, and taxpayers—to adjust their expectations and behavior. The Trustees recommend that Congress and the executive branch work closely together with a sense of urgency to address these challenges.

Source: 2019 Annual Report of the Board of Trustees of the Federal Hospital Insurance and Federal Supplementary Medical Insurance Trust Funds. April 22, 2019. Washington, D.C.: Centers for Medicare & Medicaid Services, 2–9. Available online at https://www.cms.gov/Research-Statistics-Data-and-Systems/Statistics-Trends-and-Reports/ReportsTrustFunds/Downloads/TR2019.pdf.

National Health Expenditure Fact Sheet (2019)

The Centers for Medicare and Medicaid Services issues the National Health Expenditure (NHE) Fact Sheet each year. The 2019 document summarizes spending during 2018. This series of brief, bulleted points offers an overview of the nation's actual spending on health care under Medicare, Medicaid, and private insurance over the previous year. Figures include spending by select demographic group, and the report presents limited information on health spending by state and region of the country. The report also shows spending projections through 2027. Previous years' reports as well as annual updates can be found at www.cms.gov.

Historical NHE, 2018:

- NHE grew 4.6% to $3.6 trillion in 2018, or $11,172 per person, and accounted for 17.7% of Gross Domestic Product (GDP).
- Medicare spending grew 6.4% to $750.2 billion in 2018, or 21 percent of total NHE.
- Medicaid spending grew 3.0% to $597.4 billion in 2018, or 16 percent of total NHE.
- Private health insurance spending grew 5.8% to $1,243.0 billion in 2018, or 34 percent of total NHE.
- Out-of-pocket spending grew 2.8% to $375.6 billion in 2018, or 10 percent of total NHE.
- Hospital expenditures grew 4.5% to $1,191.8 billion in 2018, slower than the 4.7% growth in 2017.
- Physician and clinical services expenditures grew 4.1% to $725.6 billion in 2018, a slower growth than the 4.7% in 2017.
- Prescription drug spending increased 2.5% to $335.0 billion in 2018, faster than the 1.4% growth in 2017.
- The largest shares of total health spending were sponsored by the federal government (28.3 percent) and the households (28.4 percent). The private business share of health spending accounted for 19.9 percent of total health care spending, state and local governments accounted for 16.5 percent, and other private revenues accounted for 6.9 percent.

For further details, see NHE Tables in the following downloads.

Projected NHE, 2018–2027:

- Under current law, national health spending is projected to grow at an average rate of 5.5 percent per year for 2018–27 and to reach nearly $6.0 trillion by 2027.

- Health spending is projected to grow 0.8 percentage point faster than Gross Domestic Product (GDP) per year over the 2018–27 period; as a result, the health share of GDP is expected to rise from 17.9 percent in 2017 to 19.4 percent by 2027.

- Key economic and demographic factors fundamental to the health sector are anticipated to be the major drivers during 2018–27.

- Prices for health care goods and services are projected to grow somewhat faster over 2018–27 (2.5 percent compared to 1.1 percent for 2014–17).

- As a result of comparatively higher projected enrollment growth, average annual spending growth in Medicare (7.4 percent) is expected to exceed that of Medicaid (5.5 percent) and private health insurance (4.8 percent).

- The Medicare enrollment impacts are the key reason the share of health care spending sponsored by federal, state, and local governments is expected to increase by 2 percentage points over the projection period, reaching 47 percent by 2027.

- The insured share of the population is expected to remain stable at around 90 percent throughout 2018–27.

  For further details, see NHE projections 2018–2027 in the following downloads.

NHE by Age Group and Gender, Selected Years 2002, 2004, 2006, 2008, 2010, 2012, and 2014:

- Per person personal health care spending for the 65 and older population was $19,098 in 2014, over five times higher than spending per child ($3,749) and almost 3 times the spending per working-age person ($7,153).

- In 2014, children accounted for approximately 24 percent of the population and about 11 percent of all PHC spending.
- The working-age group comprised the majority of spending and population in 2014, almost 54 percent and over 61 percent, respectively.
- The elderly were the smallest population group, nearly 15 percent of the population, and accounted for approximately 34 percent of all spending in 2014.
- Per person spending for females ($8,811) was 21 percent more than males ($7,272) in 2014.
- In 2014, per person spending for male children (0–18) was 9 percent more than females. However, for the working age and elderly groups, per person spending for females was 26 and 7 percent more than for males.

    For further details, see health expenditures by age in the following downloads.

NHE by State of Residence, 1991–2014:

- In 2014, per capita personal health care spending ranged from $5,982 in Utah to $11,064 in Alaska. Per capita spending in Alaska was 38 percent higher than the national average ($8,045) while spending in Utah was about 26 percent lower; they have been the lowest and highest, respectively, since 2012.
- Health care spending by region continued to exhibit considerable variation. In 2014, the New England and Mideast regions had the highest levels of total per capita personal health care spending ($10,119 and $9,370, respectively), or 26 and 16 percent higher than the national average. In contrast, the Rocky Mountain and Southwest regions had the lowest levels of total personal health care spending per capita

($6,814 and $6,978, respectively) with average spending roughly 15 percent lower than the national average.

• For 2010–14, average growth in per capita personal health care spending was highest in Alaska at 4.8 percent per year and lowest in Arizona at 1.9 percent per year (compared with average growth of 3.1 percent nationally).

• The spread between the highest and the lowest per capita personal health spending across the states has remained relatively stable over 2009–14. Accordingly, the highest per capita spending levels were 80–90 percent higher per year than the lowest per capita spending levels during the period.

• Medicare expenditures per beneficiary were highest in New Jersey ($12,614) and lowest in Montana ($8,238) in 2014.

• Medicaid expenditures per enrollee were highest in North Dakota ($12,413) and lowest in Illinois ($4,959) in 2014.

For further details, see health expenditures by state of residence in the following downloads.

NHE by State of Provider, 1980–2014:

• Between 2009 and 2014, U.S. personal health care spending grew, on average, 3.9 percent per year, with spending in North Dakota growing the fastest (6.7 percent) and spending in Rhode Island growing the slowest (2.5 percent).

• In 2014, California's personal health care spending was highest in the nation ($295.0 billion), representing 11.5 percent of total U.S. personal health care spending. Comparing historical state rankings through 2014, California consistently had the highest level of total personal health care spending, together with the highest total population in the nation. Other large states, New York, Texas, Florida, and Pennsylvania, also were among the states with the highest total personal health care spending.

• Wyoming's personal health care spending was lowest in the nation (as has been the case historically), representing just

0.2 percent of total U.S. personal health care spending in 2014. Vermont, Alaska, North Dakota, and South Dakota were also among the states with the lowest personal health care spending in both 2014 and historically. All these states have smaller populations.

- Gross Domestic Product (GDP) by state measures the value of goods and services produced in each state. Health spending as a share of a state's GDP shows the importance of the health care sector in a state's economy. As a share of GDP, Maine ranked the highest (22.3 percent) and Wyoming ranked the lowest (9.3 percent) in 2014.

Source: Centers for Medicare & Medicaid Services. Available online at https://www.cms.gov/Research-Statistics-Data -and-Systems/Statistics-Trends-and-Reports/NationalHealth ExpendData/NHE-Fact-Sheet.

GAO Report on the Medicare Advantage Plan Finder (2019)

While Medicare Advantage plans are popular, evidence indicates that seniors do not make the most efficient use of the comparative shopping opportunity they have each year during the enrollment period, and the search process is often complicated. In 2019, the Government Accountability Office studied the experiences of beneficiaries as well as professional plan navigators—the staff of State Health Insurance Assistance Programs—and found that while the professional staff members tended to not report problems with searching, seniors did. The summary of this report to Congress appears here.

The Medicare Plan Finder (MPF) website—a primary resource for comparing Medicare coverage options—is difficult for beneficiaries to use and provides incomplete information, according to stakeholders and research studies. These sources and directors of State Health Insurance Assistance Programs (SHIP)

GAO surveyed—who assist beneficiaries with their Medicare coverage choices—reported that beneficiaries struggle with using MPF because it can be difficult to find information on the website and the information can be hard to understand. For example, MPF requires navigation through multiple pages before displaying plan details, lacks prominent instructions to help beneficiaries find information, and contains complex terms that make it difficult for beneficiaries to understand information. In response to GAO's survey, 73 percent of SHIP directors reported that beneficiaries experience difficulty finding information in MPF, while 18 percent reported that SHIP counselors experience difficulty. Stakeholders and SHIP directors reported that MPF provides incomplete estimates of costs under original Medicare, making it difficult to compare original Medicare and Medicare Advantage (MA), the program's private health plan alternative. Specifically, MPF's plan results pages do not integrate information on Medigap plans. (These plans help cover some of beneficiaries' out-of-pocket costs.) Seventy-five percent of the SHIP directors surveyed reported that the lack of Medigap information in MPF limits the ability of beneficiaries to compare original Medicare to MA. The Centers for Medicare & Medicaid Services (CMS)—the agency that administers MPF—is aware of the difficulties beneficiaries face using MPF and is planning to launch a redesigned website in August 2019. According to CMS, redesigning MPF involves multiple iterations of changes and ongoing user testing, and CMS will know more about how well the redesigned MPF addresses user needs after it is used by beneficiaries.

Source: U.S. Government Accountability Office. Medicare Plan Finder: Usability Problems and Incomplete Information Create Challenges for Beneficiaries Comparing Coverage Options. GAO-19-627. July 2019. Available online at https://www.gao.gov/assets/710/700585.pdf.

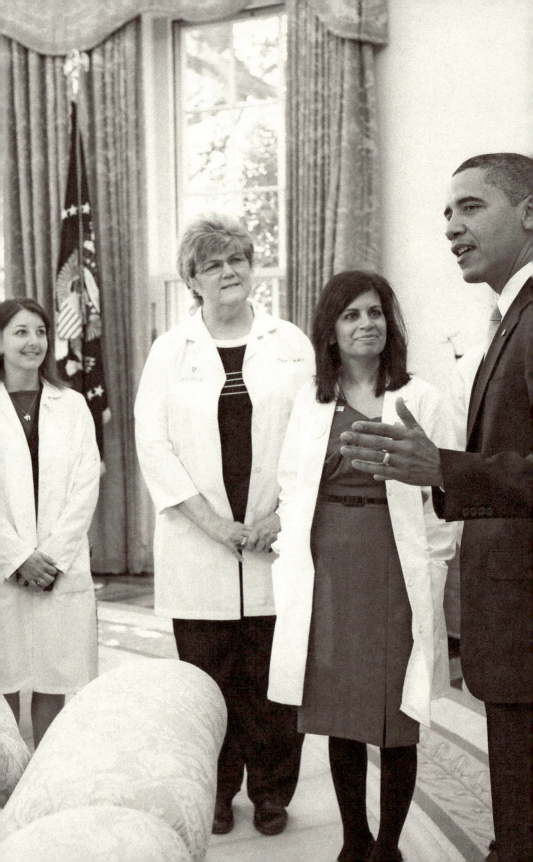

6 Resources

A vast literature has developed on health care policy in general and Medicare and Medicaid in particular. This chapter—an annotated bibliography of books, articles, and electronic documents—focuses on several areas that will help readers understand key historical developments in the life of Medicare and Medicaid. This includes both successfully enacted changes and failed efforts. The covered topics also include some of the most important areas of contemporary controversy, including managed care arrangements, prescription drug costs, and proposals to broaden these programs to cover more of the population. While Congress is unlikely to adopt Medicare for All in the near term, this idea has gained a great deal of traction among Democrats in recent years and will almost certainly continue as a prominent point of discussion. One of the following sections considers Medicare for All proposals as well as the related idea of a public option government health insurance program. The readings include works by historians, policy scholars, journalists, medical providers, policy advocates, and others.

President Barack Obama meets with medical doctors at the White House in October 2009 in an effort to rally support for the Patient Protection and Affordable Care Act, which was pending in Congress at the time. (The White House)

Broad Overviews of the Medicare and Medicaid Programs

Budrys, Grace. 2012. *Our Unsystematic Health Care System*. 3rd ed. New York: Rowman & Littlefield Publishers, Inc.

> Budrys offers an overview of American health care financing and delivery systems with an emphasis on the implementation of the Affordable Care Act. The text includes a chapter dedicated to Medicare, Medicaid, and the Children's Health Insurance Program. Allowing readers to better understand the United States in comparative perspective, the book includes a chapter on health systems in other countries, all of which have government-organized arrangements. The United States is the only developed democracy that does not have in place a system to offer health care insurance to all of its citizens. The reasons for this are many, and understanding some of this will help readers grasp the importance and very incomplete nature of government-sponsored insurance, including Medicare and Medicaid, in the United States. Budrys is professor emerita at DePaul University in Chicago.

Moon, Marilyn. 2006. *Medicare: A Policy Primer*. Washington, D.C.: Urban Institute Press.

> A fine starting point for readers interested in a broad overview of Medicare, Moon's book covers the basics of how the program works, important changes across time, and consideration of several prominent reform ideas under discussion in recent years. Of particular interest is the chapter on whether privatizing Medicare would help stabilize the program and how this would impact beneficiaries. This chapter segues into discussion of Medicare Advantage and vouchers for beneficiaries discussed in Chapter 2 of this text. Moon is a senior fellow at the Urban Institute, who has served as a trustee for the Social Security and Medicare trust funds.

Roy, Avik. 2013. *How Medicaid Fails the Poor*. New York: Encounter Books.

> This slender book has a broad agenda. As the series title indicates, this is a political broadside. Roy indicts Medicaid as an expensive program that does not serve low-income people well. The expensive part is well supported by the evidence. How to think about the quality of care that Medicaid provides beneficiaries is more complicated. Readers will come to appreciate the debate between those who envision Medicaid as a safety net versus those who would prefer to move Medicaid in a more competitive, market-based direction. Roy is a journalist and conservative policy commentator.

Smith, David, and Judith Moore. 2015. *Medicaid Politics and Policy*. 2nd ed. New York: Routledge/Taylor and Francis Group.

> A comprehensive coverage of the life of Medicaid from its creation to the present time, the 11 chapters of this text address questions of how the original framework of the program has shaped its half century of development. The text covers important amendments along the way, the funding crises associated with the program's expansion during the 1980s and 1990s, questions of federalism and state innovation under waivers, the expansion of Medicaid under the Affordable Care Act, and recent state actions with the program. The authors characterize Medicaid as a weak entitlement, which captures the fact that the program is not only welfare medicine but also a firmly ensconced part of the political landscape. This is one of the best single texts covering the life of Medicaid. Smith teaches at Swarthmore College, and Moore has been a commissioner at MACPAC, the Medicaid and CHIP Payment and Access Commission.

History

Altman, Stuart, and David Shactman. 2011. *Power, Politics, and Universal Health Care: The Inside Story of a Century-Long Battle*. Amherst, NY: Prometheus Books.

This smartly written account of the challenges faced by health care expansion advocates involves a helpful mix of history and institutional analysis that explains why the spreading of health coverage has been as spasmodic as it has been over the past century. The book is organized into four parts. The first traces the history of some of the failures of reform advocates, including Presidents Nixon and Clinton. The second discusses successful expansions, including the Hill-Burton hospital and clinic construction program of the 1950s and the passage of Medicare and Medicaid. Part three examines the rising costs of health care in private markets, and part four explains the discontent these cost increases generated and how this created the political opportunity to enact the Affordable Care Act in 2010. Readers interested in Medicare and Medicaid will find parts two and four most useful.

Catlin, Aaron, and Cathy Cowan. 2015. "History of Health Spending in the United States, 1960–2013" (November 19).
This report, written for the Centers for Medicare and Medicaid Services and available on its website, provides a detailed account of patterns of growth in health care goods and services over time. Beyond documenting the sometimes steep rises in spending, the document explains why various types of spending have risen faster at some times than at others. Readers gain an understanding of how policy reforms, especially within Medicare payment systems, have achieved some success in limiting the growth in government spending. This report makes a useful accompaniment to the National Health Expenditure Fact Sheet, which is produced by the Centers for Medicare and Medicaid Services.

Cohen, Alan, David Colby, Keith Wailoo, and Julian Zelizer, eds. 2015. *Medicare and Medicaid at 50: America's Entitlement*

Programs in the Age of Affordable Care. New York: Oxford University Press.

> This collection of contributed essays by a number of important commentators provides a historical perspective on the occasion of the 50th anniversary of Medicare and Medicaid, and it includes several incisive essays that help readers understand how the programs originated and what they have become in the intervening years. The elapsed time shows both elements of continuity and change. The collection includes chapters on Congress, the courts, states, interest groups, trends in program spending, and various other perspectives on Medicare and Medicaid. The concluding chapter addresses the formative roles played by these two programs and how they have affected America's health care system more broadly.

Funigiello, Philip. 2005. *Chronic Politics: Health Care Security from FDR to George W. Bush*. Lawrence: University of Kansas Press.

> This detailed treatment of health care politics from Roosevelt through the end of the century clearly explains the political conflicts surrounding how to best define the federal government's role in health care provision and financing. Understanding this long-running debate sheds considerable light on the evolution of Medicare and Medicaid and how they have come to be targeted at the populations they serve. The author's premise is that more progress should have been achieved, though taken as a whole the book treats the events of these seven decades in an intellectually honest and balanced way. This is one of the better histories available of the long game played by advocates for a national health care plan. The account focuses much more on the politics than on the details of policy. Funigiello is professor emeritus at the College of William and Mary.

Katz Olson, Laura. 2010. *The Politics of Medicaid*. New York: Columbia University Press.

> The opening chapters cover much of the history of Medicaid, and the later ones examine a variety of contemporary issues. Inherent in Medicaid's welfare medicine design is the conflict between the value of helping the economically vulnerable—especially children and the elderly—versus the reluctance of the federal government to fully back the program, leaving it still largely to the states. The author discusses the political instability of the program and its uncertain future in light of the program's dual identity, as one that has come to be the nation's primary way to pay for nursing home care while also being strongly associated with young families on welfare. Katz Olson is professor of political science at Lehigh University.

Marmor, Theodore. 1999. *The Politics of Medicare*. 2nd ed. New York: Aldine de Gruyter Publishing Company.

> Many health policy scholars regard Marmor's work as the authoritative history of the creation of Medicare. The author traces the complicated contours of public opinion, interest group demands—particularly the American Medical Association and other elements of organized medicine bent on opposing "socialized medicine"—and the congressional politics at a time when the Democrats were ascending and the Republicans were in the unenviable position of having lost the 1964 elections in a landslide. Marmor spells out how Medicare represented a fusion of Democratic and Republican ideas and why Medicaid emerged as incomplete as it did, based on the assumption that it would later be subsumed by a universal care program, something that never happened. Marmor is professor emeritus at Yale University.

McGuire, Thomas, Joseph Newhouse, and Anna Sinaiko. 2011. "An Economic History of Medicare Part C." *The Milbank Quarterly* 89 (2): 289–332.

This article examines the administrative and congressional politics of the creation of Medicare Part C. Designed to provide subscribers more choices and taxpayers some relief from the rising costs of Medicare, the program today known as Medicare Advantage has turned out to be very popular with beneficiaries, but it is more expensive than traditional Medicare. The question of whether Medicare Part C can both provide consumer choice and save money is the central one for these authors. The text offers some proposals for more market-oriented solutions. The authors are all health policy scholars at Harvard University.

Oberlander, Jonathan. 2003. *The Political Life of Medicare.* Chicago: University of Chicago Press.

Oberlander, a prominent health policy scholar, builds on Theodore Marmor's classic text and brings the history up to the beginning of the 21st century. This book is particularly valuable owing to how the author skillfully traces how the 1990s and the rise of conservative Republicans in Congress challenged the longstanding consensus surrounding Medicare essentially for the first time after the program was enacted. This conservative ascendency brought with it calls for more privatization. In contrast, those on the political Left pushed for a single-payer system. Oberlander highlights how the role of government provision of this enormous entitlement program drove its continued popularity, even in the face of calls for privatization from the Right. Oberlander is professor in the Department of Social Medicine, University of North Carolina, Chapel Hill.

Stevens, Robert, and Rosemary Stevens. 1974. *Welfare Medicine in America: A Case Study in Medicaid.* New York: Macmillan.

This detailed account of the creation and first decade of Medicaid includes history back to the Kerr-Mills Program enacted in 1960. The authors trace the important changes in public sentiment during that decade when the legislative discourse around medical assistance for low- and moderate-income Americans fundamentally shifted in favor of government involvement. Because states co-sponsor Medicaid, the early history of their roles and frequent resistance to expanding this program helps explain why Medicaid emerged and persisted as such a fragmented program, leaving many needy people uncovered for several decades. Readers will gain a good understanding of how Medicare was a key part of the 1960s' war on poverty.

Policy Reform Failures

Himelfarb, Richard. 1995. *Catastrophic Politics: The Rise and Fall of the Medicare Catastrophic Coverage Act of 1988.* University Park: University of Pennsylvania Press.

When Congress enacted the Medicare Catastrophic Coverage Act in 1988, it sought to extend government insurance to cover extremely costly episodes for seniors. This extended component of Medicare was to be paid for mainly by increased taxes on high-income enrollees. As it turns out, the political backlash by these wealthier seniors was intense, and other income groups did little to counterbalance the objections. Within a year and a half, the criticism heaped on members of Congress reached such a crescendo that lawmakers repealed the new program. The most interesting part of the explanation for this backtracking hinges on the dynamics of public opinion formation, specifically the framing of who would bear the costs for a program that promised to help millions of seniors. Himelfarb is a political scientist at Hofstra University.

Hirshfeld, Daniel. 1970. *The Lost Reform: The Campaign for Compulsory Health Insurance in the United States from 1932 to 1943*. Cambridge, MA: Harvard University Press.

The failure of the Roosevelt Administration and Congress to include a mandatory health insurance program under the 1935 Social Security Act has been a source of disappointment for progressive advocates for decades. Historians have long speculated that had some sort of Social Security-based program been created at that time, by now it would have evolved into a universal care arrangement. However, because Roosevelt feared that including health provisions in the pending Social Security bill would endanger its chance for congressional passage in 1935 and again in 1939, the president demurred, setting the stage for decades of political argument about the proper role of government in health care financing. Hirshfeld places most of the blame on the tactics of the movement for mandatory health insurance. Perhaps, had proponents at the time succeeded in framing this issue differently, this would have fundamentally changed the course of health politics in the United States.

Poen, Monte. 1979. *Harry S. Truman versus the Medical Lobby*. Columbia: University of Missouri Press.

Poen focuses on the Truman years and the arguments between progressives, who wanted to create a government-sponsored, universal health program, and their opponents, particularly organized medicine. This was a time when the "socialized medicine" critique was at its peak. Truman administration officials and others strongly felt that the time was still ripe to attach a health program to the Social Security Act and pushed hard for it. After this unsuccessful episode, the fight subsided somewhat through the 1950s, as progressive advocates generally settled for more incremental steps until the early 1960s. Poen has taught at the University of Northern Arizona.

Changes under the Affordable Care Act

Béland, Daniel, Philip Rocco, and Alex Waddan. 2016. *The Obamacare Wars: Federalism, State Politics, and the Affordable Care Act*. Lawrence: University Press of Kansas.

> This text skillfully examines the intergovernmental aspects of the Affordable Care Act, particularly but not exclusively the Medicaid expansion. Republican-controlled states have provided arenas for protracted fights to various components of the ACA. States lead the charge in opposing the Medicaid expansion. They have also played key roles in litigation over federal funding for the online health care exchanges, contraception funding, and the individual health insurance mandate. These authors explain how American federalism greatly complicates policy implementation, particularly in the case of Medicaid. Rocco contributes a perspective essay that is part of chapter 3.

Brill, Steven. 2015. *America's Bitter Pill: Money, Politics, Backroom Deals, and the Fight to Fix Our Broken Healthcare System*. New York: Random House.

> Brill's book is a detailed account of the creation of the Affordable Care Act and its early years of implementation. Well sourced and critical, this text helps readers understand not only the significant achievement of congressional Democrats who overcame stiff opposition to pass the law but also the significant shortcomings within the Obama Administration as it implemented this highly complex set of programs. The controversial Medicaid expansion receives particular coverage in part 3 of the text. Brill is a journalist, entrepreneur, and health care commentator.

Daschle, Tom. 2010. *Getting It Done: How Obama and Congress Finally Broke the Stalemate to Make Way for Health Care Reform*. New York: St. Martin's Press.

This insider account explains how congressional Democrats pushed through monumental resistance from organized interests to pass the Affordable Care Act, along with its Medicare and Medicaid provisions. As a former U.S. senator and lobbyist, Daschle briefly worked with the Obama Administration on health matters, and this close access to Obama allowed him to explain the twists and turns of the political process in ways that most other observers cannot. As with many insider accounts, this is a largely uncritical look at the passage of the ACA.

Government Accountability Office. 2018. "Access to Health Care for Low-Income Adults in States with and without Expanded Eligibility" (September).
As Congress's chief performance review agency, the GAO generates numerous reports, small and large, on a range of topics every year at members' and committees' requests. This one systematically examines the coverage gaps existing in states that have and have not expanded Medicaid under the ACA. Similar reports can be found online at www.gao.gov.

Hayes, Susan, Akeissa Coleman, Sara Collins, and Rachel Nuzam. 2019. "The Fiscal Case for Medicaid Expansion," report from the Commonwealth Fund (February).
This essay by researchers at the Commonwealth Fund—a nonprofit, nonpartisan think tank—briefly lays out the reasons the non-expansion states would benefit from adopting this ACA provision. Congress will still provide 90 percent of the costs for the expansion population, and this would remove a great deal of the pressure of uncompensated care costs on providers. Further, many expansion states have found ways to partially pay the extra costs with taxes on alcohol and tobacco. The essay does not consider the substantial political difficulties many Republican lawmakers would face (and have faced) in moving forward with an endorsement of a key provision of Obamacare.

McDonough, John. 2011. *Inside National Health Reform.* Berkeley: University of California Press.

> From the author's close involvement in the writing and passage of the Affordable Care Act, he explains the genesis of various provisions of the law and tells how each section of the ACA is designed to work. Unlike political memoirs, this is a dispassionate and sophisticated explanation of the ACA, including its changes to the workings of Medicare and Medicaid. This text will likely stand for years to come as one of the definitive inside accounts of the passage of the Affordable Care Act. McDonough served as Senator Edward Kennedy's chief health care policy staff member prior to the senator's death in 2009. He went on to teach at Harvard University's T.H. Chan School of Public Health.

The Washington Post Staff. 2010. *Landmark: The Inside Story of America's New Health-Care Law and What It Means for Us All.* New York: Public Affairs.

> The collective product of numerous journalists working for *The Washington Post*, this text offers a balanced and accessible explanation of many of the major provisions of the Affordable Care Act, including its changes to Medicare and Medicaid. The book is organized into three parts. The first explains the political background of how the ACA came to be. The second summarizes the law's major provisions. The third consists of excerpts of the ACA and the supplemental piece of legislation that was needed to reconcile the House and Senate versions, allowing readers to review many important parts of the statutory language for themselves in a way that is far more user-friendly than trying to read the entirety of the law.

Prescription Drug Coverage

Blum, Jonathan. 2006. "A History of Creating the Medicare Prescription Drug Benefit," report for Avalere Health.

This brief essay focuses on the congressional politics of the creation of Medicare Part D. It discussed the compromises required to win its passage, particularly on overall cost, how to deal with those individuals who are dually eligible for Medicare and Medicaid, low-income subsidies, and the involvement of private health plans. One particularly challenging task was to project consumption patterns. The awkward solution to this puzzle was to leave a coverage gap that came to be known as the doughnut hole, something the Affordable Care Act closed in 2020. Blum worked as a Senate staff member during the passage of the Medicare Modernization Act.

Congressional Budget Office. 2014. "Competition and the Cost of Medicare's Prescription Drug Program," Washington, D.C. (July).

Medicare Part D has cost taxpayers about 40 percent less than originally projected. Two main factors are to be credited for the savings. First, many existing name-brand drugs saw their patents expire, opening the possibility for less expensive generics to replace them. Second, few new name-brand drugs were introduced during this period, which helped control overall spending on prescriptions. The result is that drug spending per person only rose 2 percent annually between 2007 and 2010, compared with average annual growth of 13 percent from 1999 to 2003, the five years prior to Part C's enactment. This report further explains this pleasant surprise. The Congressional Budget Office provides nonpartisan expert analysis for members of Congress.

Congressional Budget Office. 2019. "Prices for and Spending on Specialty Drugs in Medicare Part D and Medicaid" (March).

The Congressional Budget Office, one of Congress's nonpartisan research agencies, examined recent trends in steeply rising costs for specialty drugs. These medications include Sovaldi, the very expensive but lifesaving hepatitis

C drug. While the overall expense of the Part D program has been under initial estimates, its entry into the market of a range of costly drugs in recent years will change this. Spending on specialty drugs roughly doubled between 2010 and 2015, from $4.8 billion to $9.9 billion. Updates to reports like this one will be posted at the website of the Congressional Budget Office, www.cbo.gov.

Frank, Richard, and Joseph Newhouse. 2008. "Should Drug Prices Be Negotiated under Part D of Medicare? And If So, How?" *Health Affairs* 27 (1): 33–43.

When enacted in 2003, Medicare's prescription drug benefit marked a moment both of celebration and of anxiety over its future. Since 1965, a wide variety of advocates had pushed for such a benefit, but not until the right alignment of political actors committed to its enactment, upward price pressures on drugs, and federal financing took place was this move seen as politically viable. Seniors have generally been very pleased, but observers concerned about price gouging by pharmaceutical companies complained about the lack of adequate competition, and specifically the statute's prohibition on price negotiation by HHS. While the lower-than-expected overall cost of the Part D program has taken some of the pressure off this issue through recent years, the renewed political discourse surrounding drug prices generally means this will eventually resurface as a front-burner issue. This article by Frank and Newhouse lays out the beginning of a framework for price negotiation as part of a broadly pro-market perspective. Given that some three-quarters of the program's costs are shouldered by the federal government, seniors in particular and taxpayers in general have a lot of reason to care about mechanisms that could help sustain Part D over the long term.

Lopert, Ruth, and Marilyn Moon. 2007. "Toward a Rational, Value-Based Drug Benefit for Medicare." *Health Affairs* 26 (6): 1,666–73.

In a similar vein to that pursued by Frank and Newhouse, Lopert and Moon discuss the long-term need for a way to control drug expenditures under Part D. They focus in particular on drugs purchased for individuals who are dually eligible for Medicare and Medicaid and suggest that the lower prices typically paid by the latter program should prevail in this section of the market. The authors envision price negotiation between HHS and drug companies based in part on the type of arbitration commonly used in business. Both this and the Frank and Newhouse article are predicated on the assumption that the *pro-market* should mean more price negotiation and competition, not less, even if this means allowing the federal government, the largest purchaser of prescription medications, also to play a role in exerting downward pressure on prices.

Oliver, Thomas, Philip Lee, and Helene Lipton. 2004. "A Political History of Medicare and Prescription Drug Coverage." *The Milbank Quarterly* 82 (2): 283–354.

This is an expertly written account of the politics surrounding the 2003 passage of the Medicare Modernization Act. Given that a prescription drug benefit had been advocated for decades prior to its adoption, the question of how Medicare politics finally shifted under the first George W. Bush Administration poses a fascinating puzzle for policy scholars, among others. Simplified, the answer comes in several parts: the growth in Medicare spending slowed, and this, combined with a booming economy, made the projected costs seem manageable. Further, rising prescription costs put pressures on seniors. Finally, the spread of prescription drug coverage under Medicare Advantage further whetted the appetite of Medicare enrollees more broadly for a drug benefit. Oliver is professor of health sciences at the University of Wisconsin, Madison. Lee and Lipton are emeritus faculty at the University of California, San Francisco.

Consumer-Driven Health Care

Congressional Budget Office. 2013. "A Premium Support System for Medicare: Analysis of Illustrative Options," Washington, D.C. (September).

> Over the past couple of decades, many proposals have been advanced in Congress and by interest groups that would substitute a voucher that could be used to purchase private health insurance for the guaranteed coverage of Medicare. Advocates see this as a choice-enhancing and cost-saving move. Opponents see it as a way to undermine the program. The report from the nonpartisan Congressional Budget Office presents some reference points with cost estimates and likely effects on program beneficiaries. The themes presented in this report will almost certainly continue to be the key issues into the near- to medium-term future. This and other CBO reports are available at its website.

Jost, Timothy. 2007. *Health Care at Risk: A Critique of the Consumer-Driven Movement*. Durham, NC: Duke University Press.

> Jost has marshaled an impressive array of evidence calling into question the coherency of the consumer-driven health care movement. The problem with consumer-driven health care payment systems, as he sees it, is multifaceted. Ordinary patients have neither the knowledge nor the bargaining position to act like savvy shoppers. The retail price of medical services depends heavily on the patient's form of payment. Providers face strong incentives to overutilize services. Jost shows how health care service consumption is simply not analogous to other types of market purchases. Readers will find it useful to compare Jost's text to Joseph Newhouse et al.'s book, *Free for All?* Jost is emeritus professor at the Washington and Lee University School of Law and frequent commentator on health legal issues.

Newhouse, Joseph, and the Insurance Experiment Group. 1993. *Free for All? Lessons from the Rand Health Insurance Experiment.* Cambridge, MA: Harvard University Press.

This landmark book on consumers' price sensitivity reports in detail on the largest health care financing experiment ever conducted in the United States. *Free for All?* reports the findings from an experiment that ran from the mid-1970s to the early 1980s. Its nearly 6,000 non-elderly participants were randomly assigned to one of four co-payment conditions (0, 25%, 50%, and 95%) and were observed across time to study how the varying level of co-payments affects service utilization. Broadly speaking, the authors concluded that higher co-payments indeed led to reduced service usage, though there are many qualifications to these findings. Not without criticism over the methods and interpretation, this widely cited book still stands as a gold standard study of consumer behavior in health care. Newhouse is a health economist at Harvard University.

Financing and Coverage Challenges

Aaron, Henry, and Jeanne Lambrew. 2008. *Reforming Medicare: Options, Tradeoffs, and Opportunities.* Washington, D.C.: Brookings Institution Press.

Authored by two highly experienced health policy experts, this text contains a thoughtful discussion of the nuts and bolts of Medicare and lays out a framework for understanding the politics surrounding this program. Chapters range from a primer on how the program works to program performance and discussions of specific problems, to proposals including premium support and consumer-directed Medicare. Written in a way that focuses on enduring structural concerns with Medicare, this book is still important despite the passage of time since its publication. Lambrew served in the Obama Administration as Deputy Director of the White House Office of

Health Reform. Aaron is a senior fellow at the Brookings Institution.

Blevins, Sue. 2001. *Medicare's Midlife Crisis*. Washington, D.C.: Cato Institute.

The high and rising costs of Medicare make it an especially appealing target for fiscal conservatives determined to tame the nation's largest entitlement programs. As with most publications from the libertarian-grounded Cato Institute, this text reviews the history of Medicare from creation to the early 21st century before pivoting to a discussion of what the author sees as a failure of policy makers to adequately appreciate the programs' unsustainable cost trajectory. The climax of this slim volume, in its final chapter, proposes various ways to encourage or require Medicare beneficiaries to use more of their own money to pay for their health insurance and to inject market competition into the Medicare policy space. Despite the passage of time since publication, large portions of this book still accurately reflect quite a lot of current conservative policy proposals for the program.

Cubanski, Juliette, and Tricia Neuman. 2019. "The Facts on Medicare Spending and Financing," report from the Kaiser Family Foundation (August 20).

The Kaiser Family Foundation frequently publishes briefs on public insurance program spending and coverage. This one profiles Medicare spending and revenue sources from a 2019 perspective. The KFF has produced a report similar to this one on an annual basis in recent years. Updates are likely. Cubanski and Neuman are staff members at the Kaiser Family Foundation.

Gawande, Atul. 2009. "The Cost Conundrum," *The New Yorker*, June 1, pp. 36–44.

Gawande's essay highlighted patterns of Medicare overutilization and dramatic variation in per capita expenditures across communities and states. Since this variation often exceeds a factor of two-to-one, one must ask if physicians might be servicing their patients in ways that more closely reflect local norms and the prevalence of certain specialists and their expensive technology than scientifically established best practices. As a widely read commentary written around the time of the creation of the Affordable Care Act, the essay helped prompt many conversations about the perverse incentives built into health care payment systems, including those used in Medicare and Medicaid. Gawande is a medical doctor and writer on the ethics and financing of health care.

Medicare Payment Advisory Commission. 2018. "Medicare Payment Policy," report to Congress, Washington, D.C. (March).

MedPAC is Congress's nonpartisan advisory agency on Medicare. Its authoritative reports help legislators to understand issues ranging from expenditure patterns to medical provider participation in the program, to service quality, to payment systems. It also comments frequently on new Medicare rules proposed by the Centers for Medicare and Medicaid Services to allow members of Congress and stakeholder groups to respond before such rules are implemented. This team of specialists is able to access quality data from other government offices in ways that make their documentation and analyses highly valuable to policy makers.

Medicare Trustees. 2019. Annual Report of the Boards of Trustees of the Federal Hospital Insurance and Federal Supplemental Medical Insurance Trust Funds. Washington, D.C. (April).

Published each spring, the Trustees' Report speaks to several audiences, including Congress and other policy makers, interest groups, and the general public. The executive summary is accessible to nonexperts; parts of the rest of this long report are of more interest to specialists. This document is the official annual accounting of the Medicare program and is the basis on which Congress responds to its funding challenges.

Thompson, Frank. 2012. *Medicaid Politics: Federalism, Policy Durability, and Health Reform*. Washington, D.C.: Georgetown University Press.

Much of the literature on Medicaid focuses either on the national politics surrounding the program or on the state-level decisions that shape how low-income individuals and families are treated. However, because Medicaid is a shared federal-state program, viewing it explicitly through the lens of federalism adds an important layer of understanding regarding the multiple financial and political forces at work. Thompson dedicates chapters to not only the basic federalist framework of the program (Congress funds most of it and creates broad eligibility and service coverage parameters, while the states administer it and fund the balance of the expenses) but also the often convoluted innovations undertaken via waivers that allow states to step outside of the basic federal parameters. Thompson is a faculty member at the School of Public Affairs and Administration at Rutgers University.

Recent Politics and Policy

Cassel, Christine. 2005. *Medicare Matters: What Geriatric Medicine Can Teach American Health Care*. Berkeley: University of California Press.

Because Medicare covers so many elderly Americans, and because government collection of data is so uniform under this program, analyses of Medicare spending and treatment data can be highly informative of best practices. Cassel leverages this strength to draw insights from what the program can teach medical practice more generally, in addition to discussing some of the major problems facing policy makers and beneficiaries, including the pending insolvency of Medicare's Hospital Insurance Trust Fund and difficult debates about the expensive care associated with end of life. Cassel is a medical doctor and expert on geriatric medicine. She is dean at the Kaiser Permanente School of Medicine.

Lazris, Andy. 2016. *Curing Medicare: A Doctor's View on How Our Health Care System Is Failing Older Americans and How We Can Fix It*. Ithaca, NY: Cornell University Press.

This thoughtful text written by a primary care physician sidesteps most of the ideological combat that has characterized the debate over government and health care for the past many years. Instead, Lazris asks how Medicare's expenditures could better focus on the kinds of services that would help seniors better manage their day-to-day health needs rather than offering them and their medical providers incentives to resort to expensive and overly intensive services. Readers curious about how Medicare could become more cost-effective will find this book engaging. Lazris practices medicine in Columbia, Maryland.

Mebane, Felicia. 2018. *Medicare Politics: Exploring the Roles of Media Coverage, Political Information, and Political Participation*. New York: Routledge.

Mebane analyzes the dynamics of public support for Medicare and how that is affected by changing patterns of news media coverage and participation in the program. While overwhelmingly popular, many Americans harbor deep concerns about its future and consequently generally resist reforms that would burden older Americans with cost-sharing or service reductions. This often blanket resistance to discussions of reform problematizes conversation and analysis that most observers recognize as necessary for the long-term stability of the programs. Mebane is a public health scholar at Norfolk State University, who has worked particularly on health communications.

Relman, Arnold. 2007. *A Second Opinion: Rescuing America's Health Care: A Plan for Universal Coverage Serving Patients over Profit.* New York: Century Foundation.

> This is one of many books written by medical doctors in the past couple of decades that leverages personal professional experience to propose different ways of incentivizing providers and organizing payment systems to encourage more efficient and effective treatments and cost savings. Relman's book stands as a critique of the trend of big businesses taking over the hospital sector and calls for a greater emphasis on quality care rather than large profits. He advocates for a single-payer system. Relman is professor emeritus at Harvard Medical School and is the former editor-in-chief of the *New England Journal of Medicine.*

Commentary on Proposals for a Public Option Government Insurance Program and Analyses of Medicare for All Proposals

Blahous, Charles. 2018. "The Costs of a National Single-Payer Healthcare System," a report from the Mercatus Center, George Mason University (July).

> This essay critically examines the projected costs of Senator Bernie Sanders' single-payer health care financing proposal. Readers will gain an understanding of how many questions Sanders' proposal raises, how many questions it leaves unanswered, and how dramatic a change such a shift would entail. The Mercatus Center, a free-market-oriented think tank housed at George Mason University, generates reports on a wide variety of public policy issues.

Cai, Christopher, et al. 2020. "Projected Costs of Single-Payer Healthcare Financing in the United States: A Systematic Review of Economic Analyses," *PLOS Medicine* (January).

As multiple think tanks and advocacy organizations each generate their own analyses of the projected costs of single-payer systems, various findings emerge. Some of these studies readily lend themselves to political argumentation, while others are no-nonsense economic studies. In what can be a noisy information environment, readers may benefit from this meta-analysis of studies performed on 22 separate single-payer proposals that have been conducted over 30 years. Over 80 percent of these analyses predicted net savings during the first year of operation. When the time horizon is moved to two or more years, over 90 percent of these studies projected net savings. The largest source of savings is achieved in administrative costs. The nine authors of this meta-analysis are faculty at schools of public health and medical schools.

Colton, David. 2019. *The Case for Universal Health Care.* Atlanta: Clarity Press.

As single-payer proposals proliferate, it will be easy to become lost in the details of the various plans. Colton has assembled a book-length treatment of the issues that includes an overview of the status quo, identifies problems associated with costs and coverage, and lays out the basics of what a single-payer plan would look like. This book nicely contextualizes the many other proposals readers may encounter elsewhere. Colton is affiliated with the advocacy organization, Universal Health Care NOW.

Haislmaier, Edmund, and Jamie Bryan Hall. 2019. "How 'Medicare for All' Harms Working Americans," The Heritage Foundation.

The Heritage Foundation, one of the nation's most prominent conservative study centers, has weighed in over the years on single-payer proposals and related ideas. This report, available at the Heritage website (www.heritage.org), makes the argument that a single-payer system would cost most Americans more in additional taxes than it would save them in eliminated private premiums and out-of-pocket spending. This brief report walks readers through a summary of others' analyses. Footnotes will steer readers to other publications where they can find more details.

Herzlinger, Regina, and Richard Boxer. 2019. "The Case for the Public Option over Medicare for All," *Harvard Business Review* (October).

From the perspective of those who envision medical patients as skillful shoppers, the idea of allowing Americans to compare health plans and select those that best match their needs and preferences is very appealing. Herzlinger is a prominent advocate of such consumer-driven health care plans, and here she and a colleague lay out the case that steering those in need of health insurance toward a market, albeit a government-organized market, is better than bundling everyone into a one-size-fits-all Medicare-like plan. Herzlinger teaches at the Harvard Business School, and Boxer is on the faculty at the David Geffen School of Medicine at UCLA.

Holahan, John, Linda Blumberg, Lisa Clemans-Cope, Siyabonga Ndwandwe, Matthew Buettgens, and Melissa Favreault. 2016. "The Sanders Single-Payer Health Care Plan," a report from the Urban Institute.

Owing to the prominence of the single-payer health care plan sponsored in the U.S. Senate (bill number S. 1804 in the 115th Congress) by Vermont Senator and 2020 presidential candidate Bernie Sanders, the idea of Medicare for all has gained significant traction in the past few years. As discussed in chapter 2, such a massive move would have profound implications for taxpayers, patients, the private insurance industry, employers, and others. The large cost of Medicare for All has attracted a great deal of attention, and this report from the Urban Institute—a Washington, D.C.-based, nonprofit, nonpartisan research organization—analyzes many of the issues. These analysts project that the adoption of the Sanders plan would increase federal spending by about $32 trillion over its first decade. The trade-off, of course, is that employers and families would no longer pay these funds to private insurance companies, since that market would be virtually eliminated. As the specific bills pending in Congress are amended and reintroduced over time, the particular cost estimates will change, though this 2016 report provides a good starting point for understanding many of the key issues.

Jiu, Jodi, and Christine Eibner. 2019. "National Health Spending Estimates under Medicare for All," Rand Corporation.

This study projects that aggregate health care spending would increase over its first year by 1.8 percent, using 2019 as the base year. Though brief, this report helpfully summarizes expected demand for services, changes in payment for services, drug and device expenditures, administrative costs, and out-of-pocket costs. Given the number of unknowns in this kind of study, the report also acknowledges its limitations. Although most studies of single-payer systems conclude that savings will result, and this one does not, this is still a useful starting point for readers interested in learning what questions should be asked when considering the likely costs of single payer.

Kaiser Family Foundation. 2019. "Side-by-Side Medicare for All and Public Plan Proposals."

Several Medicare for All proposals have surfaced in Congress over the past few years, and others will undoubtedly come along. The staff at the Kaiser Family Foundation have produced this side-by-side comparison document that is regularly updated. Readers can compare the overall structure of the plans, enrollment rules, benefits and cost-sharing provisions, premiums and tax credits, provider participation, financing, and more. This is a descriptive document, not one that analyzes the feasibility of legislative proposals. It can be accessed at www.kff.org.

Neuman, Tricia, Karen Pollitz, Jennifer Tolbert, Robin Rudwitz, and Wyatt Koma. 2019. "10 Key Questions on Public Option Proposals," Kaiser Family Foundation.

The idea of the federal government becoming a vendor of health insurance was entertained during the writing of the Affordable Care Act. The House of Representatives favored this approach, though the Senate did not. Since then proposals for a public option have remained part of the health care discourse among many prominent Democrats, including several candidates for president during the 2020 election season. This report, written by the staff at the Kaiser Family Foundation, guides readers through some of the key questions that such a proposal would involve. In its most basic terms, this proposal would probably involve the ability of a wide range of Americans to purchase health insurance through the online exchanges that developed under the ACA. Of critical importance would be the selling price for such policies, which could threaten to under-sell private plans, and the payment rates to medical providers, which, if low, could make these policies unappealing forms of payment. Regardless of the outcome of the 2020 elections, this issue is likely to persist so long prices on the private market continue their upward climb and millions of Americans continue to find either public programs or employer-based insurance difficult to access. This report and others on related topics can be found at www.kff.org.

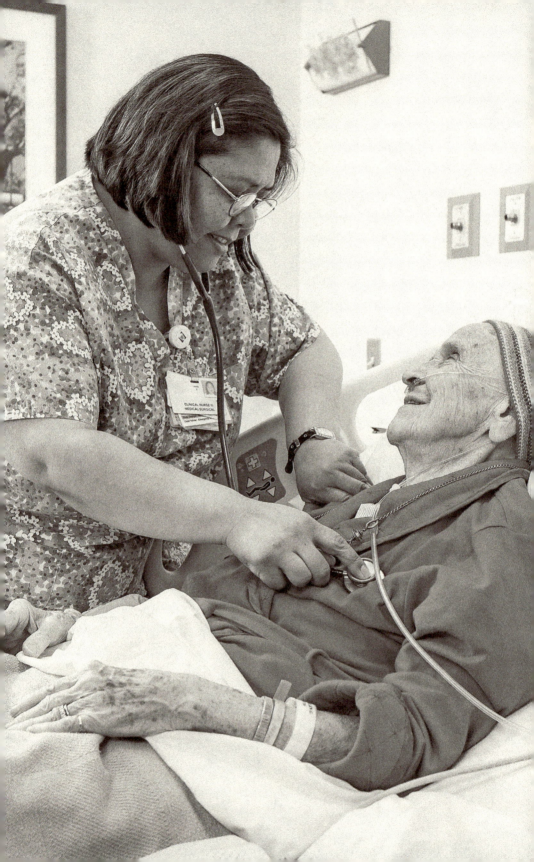

The history of Medicare and Medicaid begins in the 1930s with debates over whether or not to include federal health insurance under the 1935 Social Security Act. While health insurance was left out of that year's legislation, this prompted calls that extended over the following three decades, eventually resulting in the 1965 passage of these two large government programs. Since then, Congress has adopted numerous amendments to the Social Security Act, changing the scope of program eligibility, the services covered, the details of the funding mechanisms, and other aspects of Medicare and Medicaid. Virtually all of these changes have been incremental. The following chronology identifies many of these developments.

1935   President Franklin Roosevelt signs into law the Social Security Act (Public Law 74-271). The Act's only foray into health occurs in Title VI, which provides federal grants to states to fund public health programs (Section 602), and federal funding for research into public health, specifically studies of disease and sanitation problems (Section 603). Language in an earlier version of the bill, which is stripped out upon objections from the American Medical Association, would have allowed federal funding for research into health insurance programs.

A nurse listens to the heartbeat of an older female patient in a Medical-Surgical Care Unit in a hospital. (Philip Rink Jr./Dreamstime.com)

1950 The Social Security Act Amendments of 1950 authorize federal funds for a limited program to assist states in reimbursing medical service providers who care for low-income elderly persons. This marks the beginning of federal payments to nursing homes.

1950s Throughout the 1950s, hospital costs escalate at an average of over 6 percent per year, increasingly burdening seniors, who are becoming a larger portion of the population. These rising costs lead some Democrats in Congress to return to the idea of a compulsory Social Security-based health plan. The chief product of these discussions is the Wagner-Murray-Dingell bill, which is introduced several times during the 1950s and early 1960s.

1957 U.S. Representative Aime Forand of Rhode Island introduces a bill (HR 9467) to create a compulsory government-run health program for Social Security beneficiaries. The American Medical Association and the American Hospital Association oppose the bill.

1959 The House Ways and Means Committee hears testimony from Secretary Arthur Flemming of the Department of Health, Education, and Welfare to the effect that rising medical costs for seniors will not likely be solved with a voluntary, government-run insurance program. The Eisenhower Administration opposed a compulsory health plan. Instead, a plan is developed by Flemming and Republican members of Congress to use federal funds to subsidize purchases of health insurance for low-income seniors. Resembling the earlier Flanders-Ives bill, this is unsuccessful in Congress, but the discussions about it help foster the Kerr-Mills program, adopted the next year.

1960 The Kerr-Mills program is enacted, significantly increasing federal grants to states to enable them to reimburse medical providers who care for low-income persons. The idea of "medical indigency" is formalized as a way of labeling people who are driven into or maintained in poverty due to burdensome medical expenses. Because most states do not aggressively use this program, a small number of states account for most Kerr-Mills spending during its five-year life span. The Kerr-Mills Act also creates the Medical Assistance for the Aged program, offering financial assistance to the medically needy (nonpoor persons who face high medical costs) for the first time.

1961–1963   Congressional Democrats and members of the Kennedy Administration advocate for the passage of the King-Anderson bill, an early version of the legislation that, in 1965, becomes Medicare.

1965   The King-Anderson bill is introduced again in January. The bill works through the House Ways and Means Committee, chaired by Representative Wilbur Mills, a longtime skeptic of compulsory government-run insurance. Through the spring, it is drastically revised into Medicare (added as Title XVIII of the Social Security Act) and Medicaid (added as Title XIX) and is enacted (Public Law 89-97). In line with its focus on low-income beneficiaries, Medicaid is placed under the Social Rehabilitation Administration, an agency that focuses on anti-poverty programs.

1966   Medicare coverage begins. More than 19 million individuals are enrolled during the first year of the program.

1967   Children on Medicaid begin to receive mandatory early and periodic screening, diagnosis, and treatment services.

1968   The Moss Amendments authorize the Department of Health, Education and Welfare to withhold federal payments, including Medicare and Medicaid, from skilled nursing facilities that do not meet quality care standards.

1972   The Supplemental Security Income (SSI) program begins, creating cash benefits for persons with disabilities. Medicare is extended to persons under age 65 with long-term disabilities and end-stage renal disease. All states, except Arizona, implement Medicaid by this year.

1973   The HMO Act (Public Law 93-222) provides start-up grants to encourage the development of health maintenance organizations that will service Medicare beneficiaries who choose to enroll in managed care.

1975   The Social Security Act Amendments of 1975 create Title XX, which allows for the consolidation of social services grants to states, including home- and community-based services funded by Medicaid. This approach is appealing to policy makers because it usually costs less than housing individuals with chronic conditions in nursing homes, and it is attractive to many enrollees since they often prefer to live at or near home whenever possible.

1977   Joseph Califano, Secretary of the Department of Health, Education, and Welfare, establishes the Health Care Financing Administration to administer both the Medicaid and Medicare programs, instead of the Social Security Administration. Also, this year Congress passes the Hyde Amendment, which prohibits the use of federal Medicaid funds to pay for medically necessary abortions except when the mother's life is endangered by the pregnancy.

1980   The Social Security Disability Act of 1980 (Public Law 96-265) creates federal oversight for Medicare supplemental ("Medigap") insurance policies. Such policies become popular over the following years.

1981   States are required to provide augmented payments to hospitals that service a disproportionate share of Medicaid recipients, effectively compensating these hospitals for the low-pay work they perform. The Omnibus Budget Reconciliation Act of this year creates the 1915(b) waiver option, allowing states to pursue mandatory managed care enrollment for Medicaid beneficiaries (referred to as "freedom of choice" waivers, because they allow states to waive beneficiaries' traditional freedom of choice about their preferred medical providers).

1982   Congress passes the Tax Equity and Financial Responsibility Act (Public Law 97-248) and raises Medicare Part B premiums to cover 25 percent of program costs. This act also enhances states' ability to impose nominal cost-sharing obligations on Medicaid recipients, and it also makes it easier and appealing for privately owned health maintenance organizations to service Medicare beneficiaries. The Katie Beckett Medicaid State Plan option allows states to cover community-based services for children. (Previously Medicaid limited such payments to institutionalized children). Hospice benefits are added to Medicare. Arizona becomes the 50th state to adopt Medicaid.

1983   The Social Security Act Amendments of 1983 (Public Law 98-21) create an acute care prospective payment system for hospitals offered under Medicare, fostering greater cost control than that created by cost-based payment systems. This later develops into the money-saving Diagnostic Related Group approach with its fixed rates used for inpatient services under Medicare.

1984   Medicaid is expanded to cover children enrolled in Aid to Families with Dependent Children and pregnant women in two-parent low-income families.

1985   The Consolidated Omnibus Budget Reconciliation Act mandates Medicaid coverage for all AFDC-eligible pregnant women not previously covered.

1986   Congress passes the Emergency Medical Treatment and Active Labor Act, which requires hospitals to participate in Medicare to offer emergency services and stabilizing treatments regardless of a person's ability to pay. Also, Medicaid coverage for pregnant women and infants up to 1 year of age up to 100 percent of the federal poverty level is created as a state option.

1987   The Omnibus Reconciliation Act of 1987 gives permission to states to enroll infants up to age 1 and pregnant women in families with income up to 185 percent of the federal poverty level.

1988   Congress enacts the Medicare Catastrophic Coverage Act (Public Law 100-360), improving the coverage for hospitals and skilled nursing services, as well as an outpatient prescription drug benefit. This also creates the Qualified Medicare

Beneficiary (QMB) program, which allows the use of Medicaid funds to pay Medicare premiums for low-income persons who are eligible for both Medicare and Medicaid. States begin to be required to cover with Medicaid pregnant women and infants in families with income up to the federal poverty level. The Family Support Act of 1988 requires states to extent 12 months of Medicaid coverage to families leaving Aid to Families with Dependent Children due to increased earnings from work.

1989   Facing fierce protests from seniors, Congress repeals parts of the Medicare Catastrophic Coverage Act, including the enhancements of the Medicare payments for hospital and skilled nursing services, as well as the prescription drug benefit. The QMB remains in effect. This year Congress also expands Medicaid coverage for pregnant women and children under age six in households with income up to 133 percent of the federal poverty level. The Omnibus Budget Reconciliation Act of 1989 expands the Early and Periodic Screening, Diagnosis, and Treatment program to cover persons up to age 21 in need of diagnostic services.

1990   The Medicaid prescription drug rebate program begins. This requires drug companies to provide rebates to federal and state governments once their drugs are made available for purchase under states' Medicaid programs. These quarterly payments from drug manufacturers, referred to as "best-price rebates," are set in law and help reduce government spending on prescription drugs.

1991   Congress limits states' ability to levy provider-specific taxes and donations that had been used by states to leverage additional federal Medicaid funds (a process referred to as "bootstrapping").

1993   The Clinton Administration begins approving 1115 waivers, allowing states to experiment with innovative Medicaid projects, including managed care systems.

1995   President Bill Clinton vetoes legislation designed to convert Medicaid funding into a block grant, a move that would have ended open-ended federal funding for the program.

1996   The link between cash welfare and Medicaid is severed by the passage of the Personal Responsibility and Work Opportunity Reconciliation Act (Public Law 104-193). States are also prohibited from using federal Medicaid funds to cover nonemergency services for legal immigrants not unless these persons have lived in the United States for at least five years.

1997   Congress passes the Balanced Budget Act of 1997 (Public Law 105-33), creating the Children's Health Insurance Program. This allows states to enroll in Medicaid children who live in households with income up to 200 percent of the federal poverty level. States are also permitted to enroll Medicaid recipients into managed care programs without the state first obtaining a federal waiver to do so. Limits on disproportionate share hospitals are revised, new requirements for state Medicaid managed care programs are strengthened, and Medicaid coverage of preventative services are expanded. The Balanced Budget Act also begins a series of steps to limit future increases in payments to physicians.

1998   The website Medicare.gov is launched to provide information about the program.

1999   States are permitted to enroll into Medicaid disabled persons with income up to 250 percent of the federal poverty level. Also, this year, the U.S. Supreme Court rules in *Olmstead v. L.C.* that under certain circumstances the Americans with Disabilities Act can require states to provide less restrictive community-based services, paid for by Medicaid, to persons for whom institutional care is not appropriate.

2000   States are permitted to extend Medicaid coverage to women with cervical or breast cancer, regardless of income.

2001   The Health Care Financing Administration is renamed the Centers for Medicare and Medicaid Services.

2003   Congress enacts the Medicare Prescription Drug, Improvement, and Modernization Act (Public Law 108-173). This creates Medicare Part D and its prescription drug plan as an optional benefit for Medicare enrollees (effective 2006).

Beneficiaries with income less than 150 percent of the federal poverty level become eligible for subsidies under the new drug program. Changes to Medicare Part B mean higher income beneficiaries will pay a higher share of the premium (beginning in 2007).

2009   President Obama signs the Children's Health Insurance Program Reauthorization Act (Public Law 111-3), expanding the Children's Health Insurance Program to allow states to raise the income limits up to which states can cover children. States are permitted to enroll in Medicaid lawful immigrant children and pregnant women who have lived in the United States less than five years.

2010   The Affordable Care Act (Public Law 111-148) becomes law, calling for the expansion of Medicaid to families and individuals with income up to 138 percent of the federal poverty level. The ACA also begins to close the Medicare Part D "doughnut hole" coverage gap that had resulted from the design of the 2003 act that created the drug benefit.

2012   In its ruling in *National Federation of Independent Businesses v. Sebelius*, the U.S. Supreme Court makes the Medicaid expansion optional, instead of mandatory, for states.

2014   The Medicaid expansion takes effect. State government decisions to expand or not assume a partisan pattern, with Democrats supporting the expansion and Republicans opposing it. Over the next few years, more Republican states eventually participate in the program expansion.

2015   The Medicare Access and Children's Health Insurance Program Reauthorization Act (Public Law 114-10) changes how Medicare pays doctors, replacing the Sustainable Growth Rate method with one that encourages alternative payment models designed to boost quality and efficiency. This act also extends CHIP through fiscal year 2017.

2018   The number of Medicaid beneficiaries reaches 75 million. The Medicare program covers 44 million, or 15 percent of the U.S. population.

2020   Beginning in 2020, the Medicare Part D doughnut hole/coverage gap no longer exists. However, the standard prescription drug plan's maximum deductible increases to $435, and the catastrophic coverage range, at which point enrollees begin to receive 95 percent coverage, rises to $6,350. Medicare's high-income tax brackets are inflation-adjusted for the first time. Individuals with income over $87,000 in 2020 pay higher premiums for Parts B and D.

Glossary

This glossary emphasizes contemporary terms associated with Medicare and Medicaid. Some historic terms are also included. Because both of these forms of government insurance are laden with coverage exceptions and stipulations, a wide variety of stakeholders—including beneficiaries, medical providers, and policy makers—end up grappling with a broad vocabulary surrounding these programs. The terms included here are ones that many persons, whether users of Medicare or Medicaid or simply family members of beneficiaries, will find useful to know.

Accountable Care Organization   A network of medical providers that coordinates care with the goal of improving quality and controlling costs. Created as an option under the Affordable Care Act, ACOs are formed by a group of coordinated health care practitioners that often center on a hospital and cover patients in a specific geographic region. Medicare reimbursement to ACOs uses alternative compensation models, usually capitated (per person), payments designed to incentivize efficient and high-quality care. Groups of medical providers in an ACO can share in the savings they generate for the Medicare program.

Annual Enrollment Period   For Medicare beneficiaries, this is the period between October 15 and December 7 each year, when they can enroll in a Medicare Advantage plan.

Appeal   The process of requesting that a Medicare Advantage plan cover a product or service that it initially declined to cover. Because Medicare Advantage plans limit coverage, as do managed care plans generally, appeals are common.

Average Manufacturer Price   In state Medicaid plans, this is the average price paid by wholesaler vendors to a drug manufacturer for drugs sold at retail pharmacies. This price is used to calculate the amount of the rebate that manufacturers who participate in a state's Medicaid program are required to pay on the outpatient drugs purchased by Medicaid.

Balance Billing   The practice of a medical provider billing the patient for services that are *not* covered adequately or at all under the patient's health insurance. Neither Medicaid nor Medicare allows for balance billing.

Benefit Period   The period of time beginning the day of a hospital or skilled nursing facility admission and ending 60 days after the patient is discharged. This concept is used in measuring service usage under traditional Medicare.

Big Four   An informal reference to the four federal agencies that, unlike the Department of Health and Human Services, are permitted to bargain with drug makers over drug prices. These are the Department of Veterans Affairs, the Department of Defense, the U.S. Public Health Service, and the Coast Guard.

Boren Amendment   Federal law from 1980 to 1997 that required states to offer Medicaid payments for inpatient and nursing home care at price points that were "reasonable and adequate" to cover the cost of service delivery at a level that would meet federal and state quality and safety standards. The repeal of this provision in federal law allowed states to lower reimbursement levels to the point where Medicaid payments routinely involve a loss of money for providers.

Capitation   A fixed payment made to a managed care organization to cover the care costs on a per-person basis for a period of time, usually one year. In exchange for this payment, the managed care organization assumes all of the financial risk associated with that individual and works with its medical providers to optimize service usage efficiency. Setting such fixed payments helps to control costs. Capitation payments are used with both public and private insurance contracts and have recently become a common model for states' Medicaid programs.

Carve-Out   A term used to describe a service or a range of services that are *not* covered by a state's Medicaid managed care program, such as behavioral health services. In these instances, a state may opt to pay for such services instead on a fee-for-service basis outside of the managed care organization.

Case Mix   The distribution of patients into categories that reflect differences in the severity of illness, resource consumption, or mode of payment. Physician practices routinely set a quota on the number of Medicaid patients they allow into their case mix in order to ensure that their Medicaid patients do not outstrip their private-pay patients' ability to subsidize the financial loss associated with the former class of patients.

Catastrophic Coverage Level   The point at which a Medicare Part D beneficiary reaches the annual expense threshold ($9,719 in 2020) when 95 percent Medicare coverage begins.

Catastrophic Limit   The largest amount of money a patient would be required to pay out of pocket during a specified time period under an insurance program. The Affordable Care Act requires catastrophic limits on private insurance plans, although traditional Medicare does not offer such an out-of-pocket annual limit.

Categorically Needy   A person is categorically needy for Medicaid by having income and financial resources below a state's standard eligibility thresholds. If above these thresholds, a person might still be able to enroll in Medicaid, though he or she would be considered **Medically Needy.**

Centers for Medicare and Medicaid Services (CMS) The agency within the Department of Health and Human Services that administers Medicare, the Children's Health Insurance Program, and the online health insurance **Marketplace** established under the Affordable Care Act. The CMS also supervises states' Medicaid programs. Approximately one out of three Americans is enrolled in a CMS program. Its predecessor agency, created in 1977 when the Department of Health and Human Services was established, was the Health Care Financing Administration. The Center was renamed in 2001. The CMS is based in Baltimore, Maryland.

Certificate of Medical Necessity The document completed by a physician attesting that a Medicare patient needs and will benefit from the purchase of certain pieces of durable medical equipment. Such prior authorization is required to ensure Medicare payment.

Children's Health Insurance Program (CHIP) Created in 1997, this is an added-on module to Medicaid that allows states to extend coverage to children in households with income above the federal poverty level. Each state determines its own upper income threshold for eligibility.

Coinsurance A percentage of the cost of health care services for which a Medicare beneficiary is responsible, calculated after any co-payment has been applied. This is a form of cost sharing.

Coordination of Benefits For individuals who have more than one form of health insurance, such as a Medigap policy, this is the process of determining which policy pays first and for which services.

Co-payment A payment that an insurance plan subscriber, such as a Medicare beneficiary, must make to a medical provider, typically for each visit. Co-payments are designed to place some of the costs of services on to consumers and to cause insurance subscribers to carefully consider whether the service they might request are truly necessary. High co-payments have a marginal dampening effect on service usage.

Cost Sharing The practice of requiring an insurance enrollee (either public or private) to pay a portion of one's medical expenses out of pocket. Cost sharing can take the form of co-payments, coinsurance, and annual deductibles.

Deductible The annual amount a beneficiary is responsible to pay under traditional Medicare, Medicare Advantage, and the Part D drug program. These deductibles vary significantly by type of service. In 2019, enrollees in traditional Medicare were responsible for up to $1,364 per year for inpatient hospital services.

Diagnostic Related Group (DRG) A patient classification system that standardizes prospective payments to hospitals and encourages cost containment initiatives. Generally, a DRG payment covers all charges associated with an inpatient stay from the time of admission to discharge. The use of a fixed fee for each diagnosis, as opposed to a discrete payment for each service offered, creates an incentive for hospitals to treat patients efficiently. Congress mandated the creation of this prospective payment system in legislation enacted in 1982.

Diagnostic Related Group Outlier A patient whose condition is much more complex than normal and who consequently costs a hospital more to treat than the standard DRG category provides.

Disproportionate Share Hospital A hospital with a patient mix that is weighted toward a large portion of Medicaid patients. Medicaid's low payments create significant financial stress for such hospitals. The Centers for Medicare and Medicaid Services makes Disproportionate Share payments to states, which are then passed on to hospitals to help compensate these providers for their losses. Even after accounting for DSH payments, hospitals still experience an underpayment for these patients, though these payments help bring the Medicaid underpayment rate to approximate parity with the less dramatic Medicare underpayment rate.

Doughnut Hole   The coverage gap built into Medicare's Part D prescription drug program at its origin. At the program's beginning in 2006, beneficiaries received no government help with annual drug expenses ranging between $2,250 and $5,100, though they received assistance for drug expenses both below and above these thresholds. This gap was gradually eliminated under the Affordable Care Act.

Dual Eligible   A person who is eligible for both Medicare and Medicaid. In this instance, Medicaid funds pay the beneficiary's premium for Medicare Part B. Such a person is also known as a qualified Medicare beneficiary. Under the Affordable Care Act, Medicare became the primary insurance for these dual eligibles' prescription costs, although states are required to make payments to the federal government in order to partially compensate for the federal assumption of this financial responsibility.

Durable Medical Equipment   Devices, such as wheelchairs and oxygen concentrators, can be ordered by a physician for home use by Medicare recipients. These are durable pieces of equipment, in contrast to expendable supplies, such as hypodermic needs and glucose meter test strips. Because of the potential for abuse in the form of unnecessary expenditures, certain pieces of durable medical equipment, such as motorized wheelchairs, require prior authorization (a **Certificate of Medical Necessity**) to ensure that the purchase, to be covered by Medicare, is suitable for and will benefit the patient.

Early and Periodic Screening, Diagnosis, and Treatment EPSDT is one of the services states must offer under their Medicaid programs for persons under age 21. These services include screenings for physical or mental conditions such as hearing, vision, dental, or behavioral health concerns. EPSDT also includes treatment services to address these problems regardless of whether or not a state's Medicaid program covers such treatments for adults. Its creation in 1967 represented an expansion of services for low-income children.

Entitlement   A program that imposes a legal obligation on federal or state governments to provide services to individuals who are eligible under law. Medicare, Medicaid, and Social Security are the three most expensive federal entitlements. Eligibility for entitlements can depend on income, such as with Medicaid, or age, such as Medicare, or both, such as the Children's Health Insurance Program. Entitlement programs involve mandatory spending by the government. The more eligible individuals who apply for the program, the more the government has to spend on that program.

Exclusions   When drug plan sponsors determine which drugs and pharmacy services will *not* be covered by an insurance plan, these medications and services are referred to as exclusions.

Federally Qualified Health Center   These are community-based health care providers whose services are available on a sliding-fee scale, based on a person's ability to pay. They operate chiefly in underserved areas. As a subsidy to their budgets, FQHCs receive funds from the federal government, specifically the Health Resources and Service Administration, an office within the Department of Health and Human Services. In order to be eligible for this program these health centers must meet a set of guidelines that includes having a governing board made up mostly of local patients and demonstrating an ability to deliver high-quality, culturally competent services in ways that overcome linguistic barriers. These facilities frequently offer discounted prescription drugs and free vaccines to their clients.

Fee-for-Service   A payment system that compensates medical providers for each service, device, or supply used during treatment. Fee-for-service payment systems are widely viewed as offering an incentive to medical providers to focus on the intensity of services rather than on efficient medical care. Outpatient services under traditional Medicare are usually paid on a fee-for-service basis.

Formulary   A drug formulary is a list of prescription drugs, including both brand name and generic, that an insurance plan will cover for its subscribers. Formularies are designed with safety, cost-effectiveness, and medical efficacy in mind. These lists vary greatly across insurance plans and may specify which drugs can be covered for patients with particular conditions in specific circumstances, such as on an inpatient versus outpatient basis. Such stipulations will identify what are called formulary-preferred products. Formularies are sometimes referred to as drug lists.

Freedom of Choice   The long-standing practice that both Medicaid beneficiaries and medical providers have freedom of choice over which service providers to seek help from and which patients to accept. Freedom of choice is waived under Medicaid managed care programs, which limit the range of providers that beneficiaries can access.

Graduate Medical Education Payments   Medicare payments made to teaching hospitals to help cover the costs of medical residents' post-medical school education. Medicare is the largest provider of these payments, though most states also provide smaller payments for the same goal through their Medicaid programs.

Health Maintenance Organization   A type of insurance plan used by Medicare Advantage enrollees (as well as most persons who are privately insured) that offers a range of services within a limited network of providers. Subscribers agree to this limited access in exchange for somewhat lower premiums, and the contracted providers agree to discounted payments in exchange for a guaranteed stream of customers who are steered to them. HMOs typically limit their enrollees' range of access more than do Preferred Provider Organizations.

Hill-Burton Act   Federal Legislation passed in 1946 that provided funds to construct clinics and hospitals. This act represented a compromise between proponents of greater government involvement in health care and opponents who were suspicious of what they saw as "socialized medicine".

Home and Community-Based Services A range of services offered to the elderly and those with chronic conditions who receive support while living either in their homes or who spend time in facilities such as adult day care. These are less expensive options than are skilled nursing facilities or nursing homes. State Medicaid programs are able to leverage federal funds under 1115(c) waivers, granted by HHS, which allow them to spend funds in ways that deviate from conventional Medicaid guidelines.

Hospice Care Services designed to support patients and their families during patients' final phase of life. This care focuses on comfort and quality of life rather than curing the patient's condition. The goal of hospice care is to enable patients to be comfortable and free of pain and to enjoy each day of life as much as possible. Medicare Part A will pay for hospice provided that the attending physician documents that the patient is expected to live no longer than six months. Renewal of Medicare hospice coverage to extend the covered time is permissible.

Hospital Insurance Trust Fund The source of money for Medicare Part A.

Hyde Amendment A provision in federal law, attached to the HHS appropriations budget, that precludes the expenditure of federal Medicaid money to pay for abortions unless the pregnancy results from rape or incest or unless a physician certifies that going through with the pregnancy poses a risk to the woman's life. This provision was originally built into federal law in 1976 and was named for its chief sponsor, Republican House Representative Henry Hyde from Illinois.

Initial Enrollment Period The period when a person can initially enroll in Medicare. This period spans from three months before one's 65th birthday to three months after.

Katie Beckett Waivers A special Medicaid eligibility program for children with certain long-term disabilities or complex medical needs. This program covers in-home and other community-based care as alternatives to Medicaid services provided in hospitals or long-term nursing home facilities. Katie Beckett was a young child in the 1980s who needed such community-based services.

Kerr-Mills Program   Enacted in 1960, this program provided federal grants to states to help reimburse medical providers who cared for the indigent sick. This was a precursor to Medicaid. The legislation was sponsored by Senator Robert Kerr of Oklahoma and Representative Wilbur Mills of Arkansas.

King-Anderson Bill   Appearing in several different iterations during the early 1960s, this bill was designed to create a Social Security Act-based insurance program. In early 1965, this was amended to become the Medicare program, or Title XVIII or the Social Security Act. Its chief sponsors were Representative Cecil King of California and Senator Clinton Anderson of New Mexico.

Late Enrollment Penalty   A fee added to beneficiaries' Medicare premiums if they fail to enroll in Part D or otherwise lack appropriate drug coverage. The penalty is designed to encourage broad enrollment, which helps spread risk. The penalty is calculated by multiplying 1 percent by the "national base beneficiary premium" for Part D ($33.19 in 2019) times the number of uncovered months during which a person would have been eligible for Part D.

Look-Back   When determining Medicaid eligibility, states review applicants' pattern of having spent-down their financial resources in order to render themselves eligible for the program. Applicants are permitted to spend-down their cash savings, for instance, on routine living expenses and irrevocable funeral arrangements. Other sorts of gifts or under-compensated transfers of resources lead to a calculation to translate that given-away wealth into a time period during which the applicant will not be eligible for Medicaid. Forty-nine of the 50 states look back over 60 months prior to the date of Medicaid application. California's look-back is 30 months.

Low-Income Subsidy Also referred to as Extra Help, this program extends financial assistance to certain low-income Medicare enrollees by discounting or eliminating their premiums and their out-of-pocket drug expenses.

Managed Care An insurance arrangement involving groups of patients and medical providers bound by a contract that ensures providers a steady flow of customers in exchange for accepting lower payments for services rendered. The intent of managed care systems is to reduce overall expenditures. Medicare Advantage plans, under Part C, are managed care arrangements, though they have not been widely successful at reducing government expenditures for these Medicare enrollees.

Medicaid Expansion Under the Affordable Care Act, Congress attempted to require states to extend Medicaid eligibility to individuals and families with income up to 138 percent of the federal poverty threshold (higher for children under CHIP). In 2011, the U.S. Supreme Court ruled that this mandate was unconstitutional, a decision that made the Medicaid expansion optional for states. Since 2014, when the expansion became available, most state governments have elected to adopt this option.

Medically Needy Under Medicaid, this is an option for states that elect to help persons who have very high medical expenses and who have income above the standard eligibility thresholds. Persons certified for this help must spend-down a portion of their income during each certification period (often a calendar quarter or similar period of time) similar to an insurance deductible.

Medicare Advantage Part C of Medicare. Medicare Advantage plans are a form of private managed care insurance paid for by the Medicare program and offer patients coverage with a more limited range of providers than does traditional Medicare, but that also reduces out-of-pocket expenses.

Medicare Advantage Disenrollment   This is the period of time, ranging from January 1 to February 14, when Medicare Advantage enrollees can leave their managed care plans to return to traditional Medicare.

Medicare Buy-In   An informal term for payment made for a person's Medicare Part B premium covered by Medicaid funds on behalf of a person who is dually eligible. Alternatively, this term is also used to describe the idea of allowing middle-aged persons to purchase Medicare Part A and B coverage prior to age 65 (age 50 or 55 has been discussed). This idea has been proposed by several Democratic members of Congress since the early 1990s but has not been enacted.

Medicare+Choice   This was the initial name for Medicare Part C beginning in 1997. The name later changed to Medicare Advantage in 2003 under the Medicare Modernization Act.

Medicare Modernization Act of 2003   The federal law that created the prescription drug benefit offered under Medicare Part D.

Medicare Part A   Covers inpatient hospital services, skilled nursing facilities, and hospice care under Medicare. Enrollment in this part of Medicare is optional, but for nearly all beneficiaries (those with a 40-calendar quarter work history), this program comes at no additional cost. Part A is funded mainly by a 2.9 percent payroll tax on earnings paid by employers and employees (1.45% each) deposited into the Hospital Insurance Trust Fund. Higher-income taxpayers (income greater than $200,000/individual and $250,000/married couple) pay a higher Medicare payroll tax on earnings (2.35%). The Part A Trust Fund faces fiscal insolvency within a generation.

Medicare Part B   Covers outpatient service. Part B is funded by general revenues and beneficiary premiums. The usual monthly premium is $135.50 in 2019. Beneficiaries with incomes greater than $85,000, for individuals, or $170,000, for married couples filing jointly, pay a higher income-related monthly Part B premium, ranging from 35 to 85 percent of Part B program costs, or $189.60–$460.50 per person per month in 2019.

Medicare Part C   The part of Medicare that offers managed care plans, also called Medicare Advantage plans.

Medicare Part D   This part of Medicare offers insurance coverage for prescription drugs. Created as part of the Medicare Modernization Act of 2003, this benefit took effect in 2006. Part D is funded by general revenues, beneficiary premiums, and state payments for **Dual Eligibles**. The average Part D plan premium for 2019 was approximately $40 per month. Part D enrollees with higher incomes pay an income-related premium surcharge, using the same income thresholds used for Part B. In 2019, premium surcharges range from $12.40 to $77.40 per month for higher-income beneficiaries.

Medicare Payment Advisory Commission   A nonpartisan legislative branch agency that provides Congress with analysis and policy advice on the Medicare program.

Medicare Summary Notice   Written notices sent to Medicare beneficiaries that report services received and payments made on their behalf and that list any financial obligations for which they remain responsible. These are issued every calendar quarter.

Medigap Plans   Also called Medicare supplement insurance, these plans provide supplemental coverage to the approximately one-third of beneficiaries in traditional fee-for-service Medicare. These policies are sold by private insurance companies and fully or partially cover Part A and Part B cost-sharing requirements, including deductibles, co-payments, and coinsurance.

Noninterference Clause   This clause in the Medicare Modernization Act of 2003 prohibits the Secretary of the Department of Health and Human Services from intervening in price negotiations between drug makers and prescription drug insurance plans under Medicare Part D. This legislative language means that HHS cannot use its bulk purchasing power to negotiate lower drug prices for Medicare beneficiaries.

Original Medicare   *See* Traditional Medicare.

Out-of-Pocket Expenses   Expenses that a person pays for medical goods and services that are not covered by insurance. Medicare Advantage plans specify an annual out-of-pocket maximum amount.

Preferred Provider Organizations   An insurance plan available through Medicare Advantage that offers access to many medical providers, both in and out of network. Using out-of-network providers typically involves higher out-of-pocket costs. PPOs are more expansive than Health Maintenance Organizations.

Premium Support Model for Medicare   A concept that has been proposed but not enacted that would provide Medicare beneficiaries with a voucher that they could put toward the purchase of private health insurance instead of the guaranteed insurance coverage that Medicare has traditionally provided.

Presumptive Eligibility   An arrangement exercised by states, at their option, that allows them to speed up the delivery of services for Medicaid applicants based on their apparent financial eligibility upon application for assistance. This allows state Medicaid agencies to cover the person's medical needs prior to a formal eligibility determination. States are permitted to use presumptive eligibility for pregnant women, children, and women diagnosed with cervical or breast cancer. Other venues for these accelerated services include the Indian Health Service

Rebate   *See* Average Manufacturer Price.

Section 1115 Waiver   Under Section 1115 of the Social Security Act, the Secretary of the Department of Health and Human Services can grant state Medicaid agencies permission to implement policy innovations that "promote the objectives" of the Medicaid program but in ways that do not comply with

the standard program requirements. Imposing a work requirement on Medicaid recipients would be an example.

Shared Savings Program   *See* Accountable Care Organization.

Single State Agency Requirement   Under Medicaid law, a
single state agency must be designated to administer the program, and the program must be implemented on a state-wide
basis. This requirement ensures that no counties or sub-populations are left out of program coverage within a state.

Skilled Nursing Care   Medical treatment that must be given
or supervised by a registered nurse, such as tube feedings, complex wound care, and intravenous injections. The term *skilled
nursing facility* usually refers to a center where short-term rehabilitation services are offered, in contrast to a *nursing home*,
where residents are cared for on a long-term basis.

Special Needs Plan   A Medicare Advantage coordinated
care plan for individuals who are institutionalized, such as in
a skilled nursing facility, and who are dually eligible for Medicare and Medicaid or who have certain disabling chronic conditions, specified by the Centers for Medicare and Medicaid
Services.

Spend-Down   Under Medicaid, a spend-down is an individual's or family's income or financial resources in excess of a
state's maximum limit. In the case of financial resources, such as
bank accounts and second cars, the enrollee must spend-down
these resources on such things as medical care or customary
living expenses prior to becoming eligible for the program.
In the case of excess income, the spend-down becomes the
portion of one's monthly or annual obligation toward medical
expenses, functioning in much the way an insurance deductible works.

Spousal Impoverishment   When a person spends down
resources in order to become Medicaid eligible, commonly to
enter a nursing home, rules apply that allow the community-
based spouse to retain adequate resources so as to *not* become
impoverished.

Supplemental Insurance Trust Fund   The source of money for Medicare's two voluntary components: parts B and D.

Title XIX   The Medicaid program is found in Title XIX of the Social Security Act. Medicare is found in Title XVIII, and the Children's Health Insurance Program is written into Title XXI.

Traditional Medicare   Traditionally, Medicare has paid providers on a fee-for-service basis. The creation of Medicare managed care—initially Medicare+Choice, later Medicare Advantage—is the contrasting program. Traditional Medicare is sometimes referred to as original Medicare.

Tricare for Life   Government-sponsored health insurance for retired military service members who are also eligible for Medicare. This acts as Medigap insurance.

Two-Midnight Rule   Issued by the Centers for Medicare and Medicaid Services in 2013 and modified in 2016, this rule generally determines (with limited exceptions) whether a patient treated in a hospital is eligible for payment under Medicare Part A, which is intended to pay for what traditionally has been referred to as inpatient care. The rule states that when a patient's stay in a hospital is expected to last less than two consecutive midnights, that patient should be treated as an outpatient in the way Medicare is billed unless they meet medical necessity criteria for inpatient services. If, in the attending physician's judgment, the patient will need to remain in the hospital for two or more midnights for services determined to meet medical necessity criteria, that person can be considered and billed as an inpatient under Part A. Delivering services at an inpatient level of intensity to a person who is not being covered by Part A can be very expensive for both the patient and the hospital. Because this rule poses potential financial challenges to hospitals and patients, it has been controversial among stakeholders.

Index

About the Author

Greg M. Shaw is professor of political science at Illinois Wesleyan University. He holds a PhD from Columbia University. His research focuses on health care and welfare politics and American public opinion. He is the author of three previous books published by ABC-CLIO, *The Welfare Debate* (2007), *The Healthcare Debate* (2010), and *The Dysfunctional Politics of the Affordable Care Act* (2017). Some of his other works on American social policy have appeared in the journals *Political Research Quarterly* and *Political Science Quarterly* and other venues, including *Public Opinion Quarterly*, where, from 2008 to 2016, he served on the editorial team.